SPICY
HEALING

A Global Guide to Growing and Using

Spices for Food and Medicine

ISBN 978-0-9823570-0-2
Logos Publishing
Second, expanded edition.
Berkeley, California. 2009
Copyright © 2009 Uwe Blesching, Ph.D.
Unless other credits given, all photos are by author.
Printed in the United States of America

Table of Contents

The Great Council of Frogs

An unusual gathering was in progress – the great council of frogs had not occurred for as long as anyone could remember. They had arrived from all corners of the world - colorful, large and small, yet all glistening with tearful skins. A great sadness hung about in the air; sadness for many lost friends and relatives. A great change swept across their watery worlds, a change bringing destruction and death.

The great council debated for a long time, but when they were finished it was clear what needed to be done. A great healing was needed in the world of humans. But not just any healing, it was determined that the healing had to be safe, gentle, effective, natural, available everywhere and, most importantly, it had to be all-empowering.

The great council selected Dr. Data who had lived in a high school biology laboratory, and, who at night used the school computer and Internet to learn all about human health and healing. However, he didn't like to talk about that time at all. He had a perfect memory, never forgot anything and always ended a conversation with a question. But Dr. Data did not speak plant. So, he was not able to listen to or understand the language of the plants - nature's friendly pharmacy willing and able to partake in the great healing.

Furthermore, in order to travel to remote places of the world and learn about amazing remedies that could be used in the great healing, he needed to be able to ride the fire channels. However, he was a frog and could not do that. He could not visit even the most distant places of the world in a flash – that, only the great salamanders could do.

The great council sent a summons across the woods and into the domain of the butterflies, which are the best translators of plant known in this world. The council also sent word into the depths of the caves and crevices where the salamanders stay close to the fire channels and practice the jump - which is what they called their way of instant travel.

It was not long until their call was answered by no other than Beatrixe, the world's greatest translator of plant known to butterfly kind. From the caves and crevices and from the heat of the fire emerged Sal (yes, that is actually his name), a young and restless salamander who had mastered the fire jump when most others of his kind were still playing with tadpoles. It was said that he was as quick as a gecko and fearless like a crocodile.

The team was immediately put to task. Do you want to know what they discovered? Look for the frog, the salamander and the butterflies.

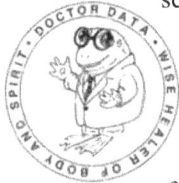

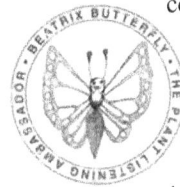

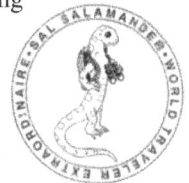

Data's comment and questions.

Sal's global discoveries.

The blue script and the yellow text next to Beatrixe are her translated voices of the plants.

Introduction

This book is written for:
- the Shamans and plant lovers who listen to the spirits of the plants;
- the science-minded lay people and health care professionals who appreciate careful study and research;
- those who believe that every illness is connected to a non-physical influence or cause;
- the men and women who like to cook with disease prevention and healing in mind; and
- those students and scholars who value a multicultural approach to dealing with illness and health.

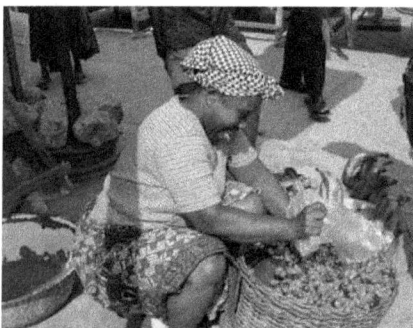

Palm kernels for sale at the Makola market in Accra, Ghana. 2008

Spices are safe, non-invasive, effective, available, affordable, natural and potentially self-empowering plant products that can be used to meet your needs for health and healing. For thousands of years, spices have been employed safely by every culture where they are cultivated or traded. They are generally non-invasive; a few of the common side effects include the burning from cayenne or the odor from garlic. Historically, global traditional medicine has effectively used spices to produce health and healing—a practice only now explored and confirmed by a body of thousands of international scientific studies. Spices are available worldwide and either are very affordable or can be grown for free from seeds. They are a natural and sustainable means to prevent or treat specific diseases.

How to Use this Book

Three cornerstones brace this book. Each can be used as a jumping off point to explore a practical use of this information for disease prevention, desired level of energy, self-exploration, health and healing. Each monogram begins with a picture and an introductory story about a particular spice. As a **first cornerstone**, you might read a bit about the assumed place of origin, the environment, a legend, myth, or ethnic fairy tale, which for the most part is a reflection of a **people's knowledge base** on how to use this plant or particular powers ascribed to it.

The **second cornerstone** underscores properties of plants that have withstood the test of time and are now being rediscovered through modern **scientific research.** This includes both globally-recognized therapeutic uses of plants and those uses confirmed or supported by modern scientific research. Research results are summarized and presented alphabetically, dependent on the region of origin. This was done, in part, to show where connections between traditional knowledge and therapeutic properties were made.

The **third cornerstone** is the body–mind connection (psychosomatics). On the first page of the monogram on each new spice you will find a section at the bottom of the page that translates the therapeutic properties of "the spirit of spices" into a form that bridges the body–mind gap. The "butterfly-plant" narrative engages the intuitive part of mind to give you a feel for the plant from the inside out. Here, properties are related to possible underlying non-physical causes of diseases. Since most spices have multiple therapeutic properties, I focused mostly on those properties that are present in all three cornerstones: **traditional knowledge, scientific research and potential psychosomatics**.

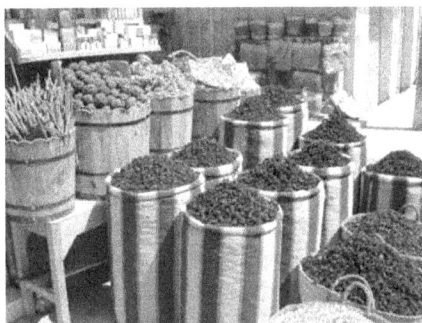

Spice display Aswan market, Egypt 2006

However, as a rule of thumb, when you are beginning self-exploration of an illness or disease, you may find it helpful to find out what the illness is keeping you from doing. Specifically, it may be necessary for you to know how you feel about this limitation so you can decipher the coded message--that is, the message the disease may hold for you. Consider using this feeling as a compass to guide you to an experience, and perhaps a belief that has been born from it. Once the feeling is expressed--appropriately and safely--ask whether this belief still holds relevance. Does it serve you in producing the emotional reality that you really want? If not, begin the process of changing the belief and engage in generating a replacement that in turn serves you better to learn, grow and evolve. You can choose a particular spice as a sensual bridge to enhance and stimulate the crossing into a more healthy reality.

In the last section of this book, I have written a guide to the information from these three cornerstones, and rather than presenting a traditional index, I have created an easy-to-use chart that shows the correlation between the spices and their potential therapeutic uses. You can use them in cooking to develop a regimen to promote health and prevent disease, as a catalyst for a desired level of energy, or for renewed health and healing in general.

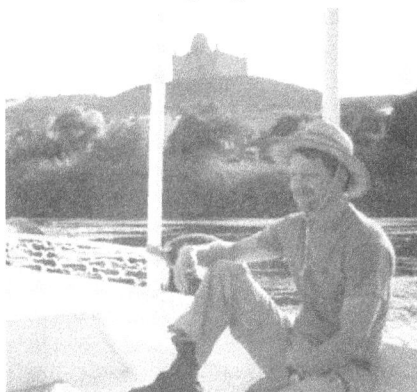

Author on Nile ferry, Aswan. Egypt 2006
Photo by Christel Blesching

Author's Note

I have come to believe that all illness originates in the mind and that the healing of anything can be more effective and permanent if it inclusively involves and connects the body, mind and spirit. Clearly this triadic interaction exists--few would argue the contrary. Consider the positive impact of exercise and good nutrition and the negative effects of smoking and fast foods.

In addition, to varying degrees, most healthcare practitioners acknowledge that constant states of fear, anxiety, guilt and harbored anger negatively impact biological bodily functions and psychological attitudes.

Have you ever experienced a disconnect from the world and felt cynical, alone, pessimistic, afraid or hopeless. What has been the negative effect on your body, mind or spirit?

By the same token, when we have a strong sense of a connection with something larger than our physical selves, all is well. An affinity is a natural connection. Each of us possesses some affinity for the smell or taste of a particular spice. That affinity is a connection to the healing spirit of a spice, which we can employ for our own health and healing.

A Brief History of Known Ancient "Spice Cultures"

The use of spices for health and healing remains somewhat obscured in the modern world. Still, the true connection has never been fully severed. It is said that if you want to hide something - put it into plain view. Today, life has put spices in plain view. Due in part to availability and price, they are usually found in kitchen cabinets everywhere. Primarily, people use spices for their culinary enhancement and delight while ignoring their hidden powers and abilities, which lay waiting to be re-discovered.

In another time and place spices and their secrets were more valuable and guarded than gold. I believe that it is quite possible that European monarchs knew more about the value of spices than has been suggested by most current history books.

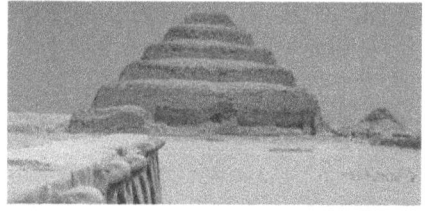

Step pyramid in Saqqara, Egypt 2006

Perhaps royalty did not just fund the wicked and gruesome invasions of Africa in search for slaves, gold or diamonds. Perhaps the promise of ancient mysteries enticed some of these men and women. They may have ventured to that continent in search of the knowledge that gave rise to the architecture of the pyramids or the temple of Karnak, to formulas for higher mathematics, astronomy, astrology, geography, geodesy, art and philosophy, and to the mysteries behind religion, physics, chemistry, education, agriculture, and, of course, medicine. Did they search for the elusive fountain of youth, increased sexual virility, esoteric powers or abilities, or possible cures to the many plagues of the time?

Ancient religious texts, historical records, medical treatises, myths and legends tell us these early civilizations sought to heal, and sought to be free of physical ailments and related mental states of feeling disconnected, alone and hopeless. They observed the impact of these emotions on the body, mind and spirit. They too searched to find healthy ways to express anger and fear. The people of Sumeria, Nubia, Egypt and India each shared similar creation myths that included: freedom from pain, fear and death, interplanetary collisions, the formation and destruction of planets, alien gods that created mankind, alien visitations, flight by "magic" means, star religions, wars conducted in the name of different gods, deities mating with humans, an immaculate conception, demi-gods, an eventual return, a flood, prophesies, kingships, immortality, extreme longevity, a paradise, a fountain of youth, an elixir of life, gifts of magical plants and spices for food, transcendence, health and healing.

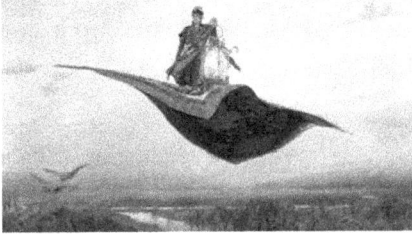

Viktor Vasnetsov. The flying carpet (1880) Russia.

Since time immemorial these records have revealed the mysteries of spices. These edible items have the ability to connect--to enable one to talk with "the spirit," thus to diminish pain, alleviate suffering, produce longevity, increase virility, and assist in producing an environment in which the body can return to complete health or regenerate itself, like the mythical phoenix that employed myrrh, a scent spice, to achieve extreme longevity and perhaps even immortality.

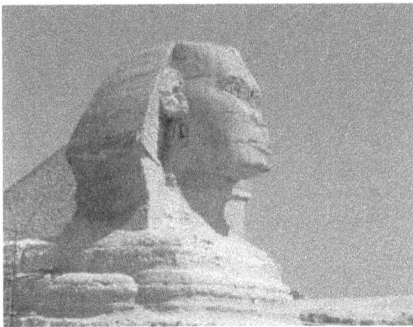

The Sphinx, Cairo 2006

Every major religion's holy book contains some form of witness accounts of spices' healing powers. Ancient texts, such as the Bible, the Qu'ran, Egyptian papyrus scrolls, and Sumerian and Mesopotamian clay tablets include historical references to the miraculous and medicinal uses of spices.

Historical texts from the Sumerian, Nubian and Egyptian, and Indus Valley civilizations echo similar reports. We hear of the food of the Gods, the white powder of gold, and the golden tear from the eye of Horus. Thoth, Enoch and Hermes Trisgetimus (three different names but perhaps the same person or character) achieved immortality and were taken to the heavenly abode without dying.

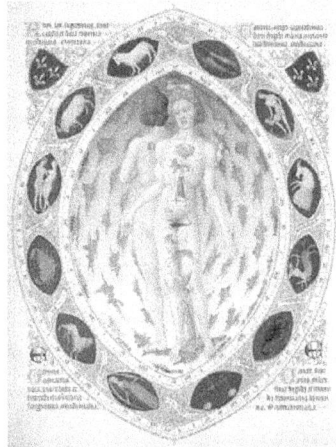

Les Très Riches Heures du duc de Berry. Anatomical Man. 15th Century, France

However, it was not just extreme longevity that was bestowed by the edible gifts of the gods. These "plant" items also yielded certain powers: telepathy, teleportation, levitation, the ability to talk directly with God and the ability to know when someone is lying.

More than one thousand years ago,

Ibn Sina (aka, Avicenna), the Persian Muslim scientist, wrote *The Canon of Medicine*, a famous and practical medical text. This 14-volume encyclopedia covers the basics of ancient Persian and Arabian medical knowledge. To this day, it is considered one of the most famous texts in the history of medicine. Until the 18th century, it stood as the cornerstone for the physician education in Europe and Arabia. Several of its principles remain relevant today. Ibn Sina wrote extensively about the connections between the emotions and physical health, and about the uses of nearly 700 plant-based drugs.

It is no accident that the historical trade in legends, myths, knowledge, herbs, minerals, animal products and spices has become a colorful mix of the same qualities they contain. For instance, exotic spices and the well-kept secret knowledge on how to use them (specifically, to advance one's desires) may have been the reason for their high value. And, this may be why the most valuable items carried on the caravans traversing the lands from the Far East to the shores of Europe were so incredibly expensive. Only the richest could afford items that were deemed by so many to be so powerful and important to our life and well-being.

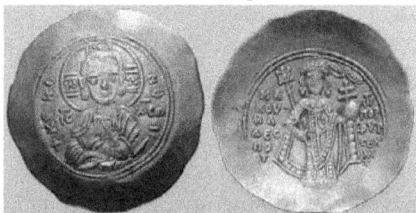

12th century gold coin of Byzantine Emperor
Courtesy: CNG Coins

But, that was then, and this is now. This is the day of the Internet and the time of the global citizen. Spices, which are pretty much available anywhere, tend to be universally inexpensive. For centuries, numerous plants have been used to prevent illness or help obtain better health, youthfulness, and virility, and to gain access to esoteric resources. Each of these plants discussed in this book has a well-established time-proven record. Each of them has been dissected and explored extensively by modern scientific research. When you add your own experience and affinity to this plethora of information presented here you can further personalize your experience and exploration of these spices, resulting in a practical guide for your own specific health and healing needs.

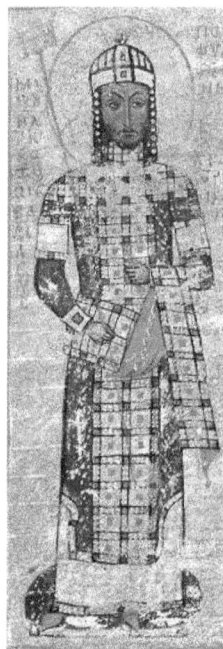

Manuel Comnenus was one of the Byzantine Emperors whose riches were based largely on spice and silk. Courtesy: Adam Bishop

1 McCallum, M. L. *Amphibian Decline or Extinction? Current Declines Dwarf Background Extinction Rate.* Journal of Herpetology. 41(3):483–491. 2007.

For my mother and my sister

two constant sources of support in my universe

Acknowledgement

I wish to acknowledge Tim Sunderman for his help with the layout, graphics and creation of the cover art; Ellen Mulholland for text editing the project; A. Kim for her support throughout the writing of this project; David and Chris Elise Anderson for their general creative input; Elsa Gebreamlak for her assistance in translating Amharic research text into English; John Bilorusky, Ph.D., for unique insights into action research methodology; media consultant Humphrey Jojo Quayson, Ghana; Retired Major Quarshigah, the Minister of Health, Ghana; Mr. Arhin and Dr. Agyemfra from the Traditional Alternative Medicine Directorate (TAMD), Ministry of Health, Ghana; Professor Okine, Mr. Archibald and Pharmacologist Osafo-Mensah from the Centre for Scientific Research into Plant Medicine, Mampong, Ghana; Paul Ntima and Samuel Essilfie - traditional bonesetters at the Aponche Memorial Herbal Clinic; David Chick Forkam at the Limbe Botanical Gardens, Cameroon; former U.S. Representative of California, Ronald Dellums and his staff for assistance in dealing with the State Department to obtain the permit to frequent travels to Cuba; Alfredo Naranjo M.D., Pediatric Cardiac Surgeon; acupuncturist Dr. Rafael Chiong Molina and Daura Garcia Sagado, Havana, Cuba with whose assistance I was able to better understand the strengths and weaknesses of the Cuban health care delivery system; and, an old friend who likes to remain anonymous.

Disclaimer

This text is a compilation of knowledge. I have made a very strong effort to assure accuracy by double-checking and cross-referencing this knowledge with other scientific literature and credible documented evidence. However, I cannot guarantee that the information herein contained holds up to the differences in opinion of other health care professionals and organizations. Further, the possibility exists that some of the information in this book contains human error.

This book is not intended as a guide for self-treatment or self-medication. The lay reader is strongly advised to work closely with the legally authorized health care professional of his or her choice when considering any information contained herein.

Neither the authors, editors or publishers accept any responsibility for the accuracy of the information itself or the consequences from the use or misuse of the information presented in this book, or excerpts from it in any other form of publication.

Consider, that through the beliefs you hold and the choices you make based on them, you are ultimately responsible for your energy, your well-being, your healing or the lack of it.

Key to Text Icons

Important quetions   Global discoveries   Herb talks

Worlds of Healing

Acacia

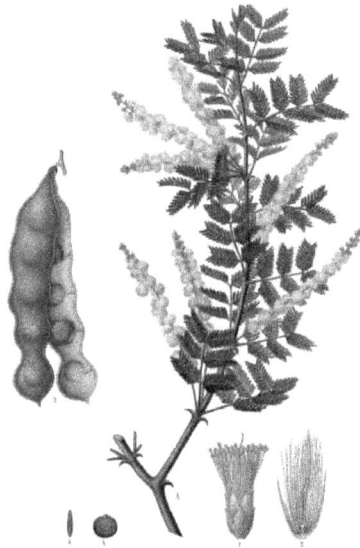

Acacia Senegal, Köhler's Medicinal Plants 1887

Return, return
from bitterness
to the sweetness
of life.

Whatever the Arc of the Covenant actually was - 'a container for the broken stone tablets written by god,' 'a weapon' (able to destroy the walls of Jericho), or 'a mysterious device capable of levitation and lightening' — we may never know, but it is written, it was fashioned from gold-plated acacia (Shittim) wood.

The story of the biblical drama in which acacia plays its part begins with Moses who went upon the mount to stand before God. When the people of Israel saw that Moses, their "go-between", did not return as quickly as they wished, the Israelites said 'anxiously' to Aaron in their apparent desire to also be before God: "Up, make us gods, which shall go before us; ..." 'And Aaron (arc means aron in Hebrew) collected their gold earrings, melted

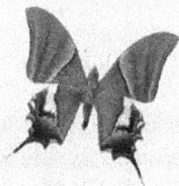

My gum, leaves and powdered pods have the ability to nurture you, to ease your fears; and I can help you realize that you can cope with what you fear. I can ease your soreness and help release your irritation by bringing calm and peace into your mind. I can help return you from bitterness to the sweetness of life.

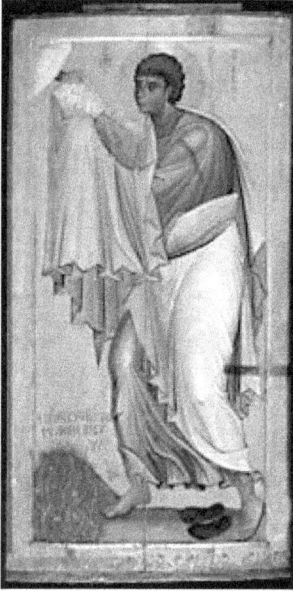

Moses receiving the law. Getty Center. Unknown artist ca. 1050-1100

Egyptologist, who found 'tons of it' in 1904 at a 'temple-mount' in Sinai. Apparently, it was mentioned in many hieroglyphs and was translated as mfkzt. A white powder with similar esoteric properties has been called shem-an-na in Mesopotamian texts, the tear of Horus in Egypt, the Golden Fleece in Greece, and the 'food of the gods'. Myths talk of its ability to gift telepathy, 'be before god', and allow longevity, evolution, healing, and spiritual revitalization. (see Moses and the golden calf).

Although, acacia gum, a fine white powder, may not be the mysterious mfkzt; one of acacia's known medicinal properties is its ability to enhance relaxed states, reduce anxiety and function as a mood elevator. And, these are just some of what the Israelites of old

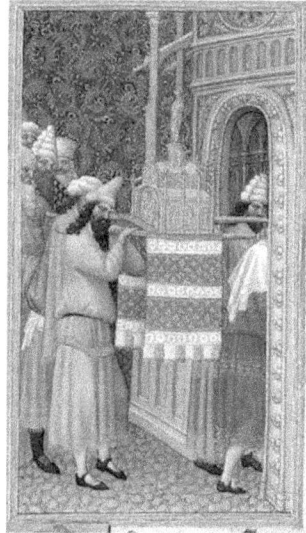

Très Riches Heures du Duc de Berry. The Ark of God Carried into the Temple the Musée Condé, Chantilly. 15th Century.

them, created the form of a calf, turned it into a statue and proclaimed': "These be thy gods, O Israel, which brought thee up out of the land Egypt."

Now the Old Testament God tells Moses that the Israelites "had corrupted themselves" and had somehow gotten 'it' wrong. To right this 'wrong' Moses climbed down from the mount: "And he took the calf (golden) which they had made, and burnt it in the fire, and ground it to powder, and strawed it upon the water, and made the children of Israel drink of it." The powdered 'gold' was used to 'heal the spiritually corrupted'.

Other legends that contain claims of similar nature are that of alchemy, the philosopher's stone that can turn lead (the ordinary person) into gold ('enlightened person'). A mysterious white powder, perhaps also obtained from 'burning' gold, has been recorded by Sir William Flinders Petrie, the British

seemed to have been looking for when they were asking Aaron for help.

To this day acacia is one of the main symbols in Freemasonry and can be seen in the emblem of the Masonic

Acacia Fraternity. History connects Masons with the Knights Templar, and both claim connection to the Temple of Solomon, which housed the very ark.

Acacia trees are also the symbol of Al-Uzza, the Arabian goddess and founding mother of Mohammed's tribe. It is said that meteorites are her sacred stones, which is why they are revered as the holy of holiest in Mecca.

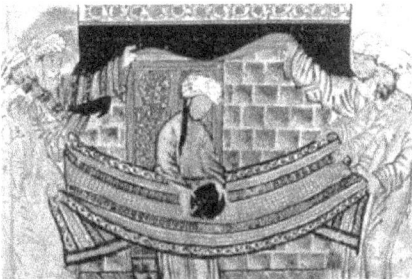

Jami' al-Tavarikh 1315. 'The Prophet Muhammad solves dispute over sacred black stone.' Edinburgh University Library, Special Collections and Archives. Out of respect for Islam the Prophet's face has been blurred.

Acacia gum or gum arabica, usually made from Acaia Senegal, was used in ancient times in the process of mummification and has been found in the ink of ancient hieroglyphics. Tannins in the plant are still used in the production of some ink today. While not a typical spice it was traded along side myrrh and frankincense for as long as anyone can remember.

Acacia nilotica trees are native to the continent of Africa, the Arabian Peninsula, Western Asia (Iran, Iraq, Israel, Syria), India, Nepal and Pakistan. However, in Australia, nonnative Acacia trees are regarded as one of the worst weeds because of their invasiveness. A healthy tree can produce more than one hundred thousand viable seeds every year.

After the rainy season the acacia gum spontaneously oozes from the trunk and main branches. This is the beginning of the gum harvest. Making small cuts in the bark of the tree stimulates gum flow. The gum runs down the cut and forms tear-shaped drops, which dry and harden in the air and are mostly hand-collected. The gum, further dried and ground into a fine powder, is today mainly used industrially as a food stabilizer, preservative and food additive. You will also find it listed in many prescriptions and over the counter drugs.

Acacia gum, comprised of soluble fiber, has the simultaneous presence of water-friendly carbohydrate and water-rejecting proteins that produce its sought after emulsification and stabilization properties. Soluble fiber is not digested by the small intestines but fermented in the large intestines producing short chain fatty acids such as acetic acid with important health properties. Once ingested the acacia-body interaction speeds up oral rehydration and functions as a probiotic food for beneficial bacteria in the intestines. The leaves of acacia nilotica, like many other acacia species, also contain some psychoactive alkaloid (DMT is the most prevalent). Could this explain its reported mood altering properties?

The following information is based on acacia nilotica research:

Parts used: Gum, leaves, flowers, roots, fruit, shoots and seed pods.

Global summary:
Used to treat: Bleeding gums and sore throats, laryngitis, sore nipples, skin problems such as eczema, inflammations, wounds, bacterial infections such as conjunctivitis, vaginitis, urinary tract infections, bacterial-based sexually transmit-

ted diseases (STD's)[2] such as gonorrhea, diarrhea, irritable bowel syndrome (IBS), parasites, cough, hemorrhoids, pain, and weight loss. Additionally, acacia can reduce the occurrences of carbohydrate induced diseases or complications such as in adult onset diabetes for example.

Used as a(n): Nutritious, anti-inflammatory, liver-protective, anti-bacterial, cancer-protective, anti-oxidant, antithelmintic (destroys worms), anti-catarrhal (loosens phlegm), anti-fungal, antimalarial, astringent (tissue constricting), hemostatic, analgesic, diuretic, blood pressure (extract of pods)[1] and anxiety reducing and mood elevator (flowers and leaves).

Ancient Egypt:

The Ebers papyrus, an ancient Egyptian medical scripture describes the use of acacia in the treatment of worms, hemorrhoids, diarrhea, birth control, internal bleeding and in the care of skin diseases. Egyptians and Arabic physicians used acacia gum as a pain-reliever base. They applied it to open wounds as a cover and an antiseptic. The gum supported loose teeth, while the astringent properties of the acacia worked to tighten the surrounding tissue. Often the tooth could be saved in this manner. Acacia gum and leaves treated coughs in ancient times. The gum was also part of a remedy to treat burns to the skin.

Nubian Egypt:

Nubians in the upper Nile Valley call acacia trees Gurti. They use all parts of the tree. Nubians have found a variety of uses: mixed into a sitz-bath after the delivery of a baby to disinfect and to reduce blood flow; to treat diabetes; and, to balance carbohydrate eating with the use of powdered pods.

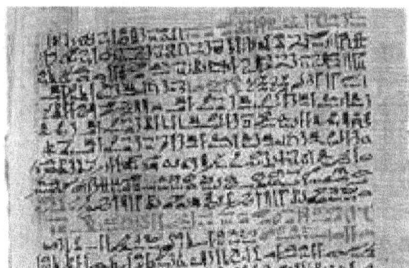

Ebers papyrus. Courtesy: U. S. National Medical Library at the National Institutes of Health

Zulu - South Africa:

Zulu traditional healers use acacia for a variety of ailments: to loosen phlegm; and, to heal inflammations of the mucus membranes.

Summary medicinal properties supported by scientific studies:

Anti-hypertensive, antispasmodic, antibacterial (STD's), anti-viral, general stimulant and mood enhancer, stool consistency (helps with both diarrhea and constipation), liver protective, anticancer and anti-mutagenic.

Egypt - Asyut:

Only date palms outnumber Acacia trees along the shores of the Nile. A veterinary study using goats from Egypt found that the more acacia leaves the goats were eating, the less bacteria found in their fecal samples - indicating an antibacterial mechanism in acacia.[3]

India - Jaipur:

Another animal study from India found anti-tumor properties[4] in acacia, suggesting possible cancer preventative abilities. Ayurvedic practitioners have long used acacia to rid the body of worms and parasites, treat wounds, nose bleeds (powdered gum), sore nipples, as food for diabetics (since it does not convert into sugar), and for the treatment of coughs. A study from Mumbai, presented at the 8th International Congress on Drug Therapy in HIV Infection, indicated that the aqueous extract of acacia pods as effective in-vitro against the viral enzyme reverse transcriptase.[5]

Kenya - Masai:

The Masai call acacia nilotica 'olkiloriti', and a UNESCO sponsored study found acacia to be the most frequently used soup plant. The root or stem bark is boiled in water and the decoction drunk alone or added to soup.[6] The moran, young circumcised unmarried Masai men, apparently prefer taking acacia leaves as a stimulant before going on hunts. This may be due to the psychoactive compound DMT found in the acacia leaf.

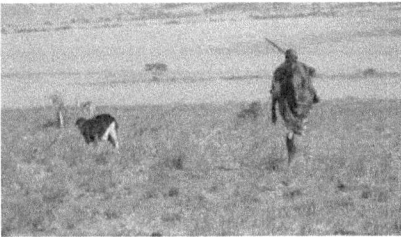

Masai hunter, Eastern Serengeti, 2006
Courtesy: Steve Pastor.

Saudi Arabia - Riyadh:

Scientists from Riyadh have found in animal models that gum Arabic/acacia has a strong protective effect when given five days prior to exposure to acetaminophen overdoses, which normally result in liver failure and death.[7] Furthermore, another study suggests that gum Arabic/acacia contains cardio-protective properties by the means of superoxide scavengers, potent antioxidants.[8]

United States - New York:

This study suggests that gum Arabic/acacia improves intestinal absorption in the cases of infant diarrhea.[9]

United States - Minneapolis:

Acacia improves stool consistency and reduces the occurrence of fecal incontinence[10] in adults. Some alternative practitioners in the U.S. have begun to use the highly soluble fiber to ease symptoms of irritable bowel syndrome (IBS). Further studies are under way to determine the mechanism whereby acacia appears to reduce sugar-induced weight gain.

Preparations used in Nubia[11]:

Nubians prepare the bath water by using the acacia leaves. They are boiled for about 10 minutes and allowed to soak for another twenty minutes. The water is used to treat gum inflammations by gargling and for vaginal baths after delivery.

To treat diarrhea or to reduce a fever, Nubians make a tea from the gum, leaves or shoots of the tree. Consume up to three cups throughout the day.

Nubian herbalists treat diabetes with a teaspoon of powdered acacia pods taken on an empty stomach. It is also used to balance carbohydrate intakes.

Warning:

Allergies against gum acacia have been noted to cause skin irritation, swelling of the mucus membranes, asthma and anaphylaxis.

The leaf also contain a psychoactive compound called DMT and depending on dose may produce altered states. A search in the relevant literature does not indicate DMT leaf concentration.

Possible interaction with drugs:

Acacia gum may also reduce the rate of the absorption of medications taken by mouth.

1 Gilani AH, Shaheen F, Zaman M, Janbaz KH, Shah BH, Akhtar MS. *Studies on antihypertensive and antispasmodic activities of methanol extract of Acacia nilotica pods*. Department of Physiology and Pharmacology, The Aga Khan University Medical College, Karachi 47800, Pakistan. Phytother Res. 1999 Dec;13(8):665-9.

> Amharic: Cheba
>
> Dutch: Echte acacia, Arabische gom
>
> French: Acacia d'Arabie
>
> German: Nil Akazie – Gummi akazie
>
> Hebrew (ancient): Shittah
>
> Hindi: Babul (bark)
>
> Homeopathic: Acacia dealbata
>   (Acac-d.)
>
> Italian: Acacia d'Egitto
>
> Latin: Acacia nilotica
>
> Masai: Olkiloriti
>
> Nubia: Gurti
>
> Sanskrit: Babbulaka
>
> Spanish: Acacia
>
> Tigrinya: Chea

2 Kambizi L, Afolayan AJ. *An ethnobotanical study of plants used for the treatment of sexually transmitted diseases (njovhera) in Guruve District, Zimbabwe*. Department of Botany, University of Fort Hare, Alice 5700, South Africa. J Ethnopharmacol. 2001 Sep;77(1):5-9.

3 Sotohy SA, Sayed AN, Ahmed MM. *Effect of tannin-rich plant (Acacia nilotica) on some nutritional and bacteriological parameters in goats*. Department of Animal Hygiene, Faculty of Veterinary Medicine, Assiut University. Dtsch Tierarztl Wochenschr. 1997 Oct;104(10):432-5.

4 Meena PD, Kaushik P, Shukla S, Soni AK, Kumar M, Kumar A. *Anticancer and Antimutagenic Properties of Acacia nilotica (Linn.) on 7,12-Dimethylbenz(a)anthracene-induced Skin Papillomagenesis in Swiss Albino Mice*. Radiation and Cancer Biology Laboratory, Department of Zoology, University of Rajasthan, Jaipur-302 004, India. Asian Pac J Cancer Prev. 2006 Oct-Dec;7(4):627-32.

5 Tabassum A Khan, Pratima A Tatke, Satish Y Gabhe. *Evaluation of Aqueous Extract of Babool Pods for in Vitro Anti-HIV Activity*. Pharmacy, C.U. Shah College of Pharmacy, Mumbai, Maharashtra, India. Int Cong Drug Therapy HIV 2006 Nov 12-16;8: Abstract No. P399.

6 Maundu, P., Berger, D.J., ole Saitabau, C., Nasieku, J., Kipelian, M., Mathenge, S.G., Morimoto, Y., Höft, R. 2001. *Ethnobotany of the Loita Maasai: Towards Community Management of the Forest of the Lost Child - Experiences from the Loita Ethnobotany Project*. People and Plants working paper 8. UNESCO, Paris

7 Gamal el-din AM, Mostafa AM, Al-Shabanah OA, Al-Bekairi AM, Nagi MN. *Protective effect of arabic gum against acetaminophen-induced hepatotoxicity in mice*. Department of Pharmacology, College of Pharmacy, King Saud University, PO Box 2457, Riyadh 11451, Saudi Arabia. Pharmacol Res. 2003 Dec;48(6):631-5.

8 Abd-Allah AR, Al-Majed AA, Mostafa AM, Al-Shabanah OA, Din AG, Nagi MN. *Protective effect of arabic gum against cardiotoxicity induced by doxorubicin in mice: a possible mechanism of protection*. Department of Pharmacology, College of Pharmacy, King Saud University, P O Box 2457, Riyadh 11451, Saudi Arabia. J Biochem Mol Toxicol. 2002;16(5):254-9.

9 Codipilly CN, Teichberg S, Wapnir RA. *Enhancement of absorption by gum arabic in a model of gastrointestinal dysfunction*. Division of Neonatal/Perinatal Medicine, Schneider Children's Hospital at North Shore, The Feinstein Institute for Medical Research, North Shore-Long Island Jewish Health System, Manhasset, NY 11030, USA. J Am Coll Nutr. 2006 Aug;25(4):307-12.

10 Bliss DZ, Jung HJ, Savik K, Lowry A, LeMoine M, Jensen L, Werner C, Schaffer K. *Supplementation with dietary fiber improves fecal incontinence*. School of Nursing, University of Minnesota, Minneapolis 55455, USA. Nurs Res. 2001 Jul-Aug;50(4):203-13.

11 Moursi, Hanifa. *Heilpflanzen im Land der Pharaonen: Ägyptisch – Nubische Volksmedizin*. 1993. Institut für Pharmacologie der Veterinär Medizinischen Fakultät der Universität Kairo.

Growth: Acacia (nilotica) is an evergreen and very thorny tree that can grow between 10 - 20 meters high.

Native to: Africa, but also found in the Caribbean, the Middle East, India and Australia.

How to grow acacia: Take the seed fresh or old and boil it for about an hour. Allow to cool over night. Remove floating or broken seeds and plant directly where you want to grow. Between 1 week to 3 months you will know if the seed has germinated or not. It has been noted that the tree self-germinates more quickly after a forest fire. Tree planters who have used this observation and pre-treated the seeds with smoke noticed a higher success rate of germination. Another method is to injure the seed into growth action. Cut with a knife or use a file to scrape off part of its protective mantle before planting. Young plants are fragile, but require no maintenance once established. Plants are considered a serious pest in South Africa and Australia.

Time to seed: Anytime where the climate and soil exists to support the species. The seeds fall and self-germinate, or they may lay dormant for years waiting for a signal to wake them into growing.

Sun: Bright sun, no shade. Very drought resistant once established.

Zone: 9-11; frost sensitive when young.

Soil: Grows best in dry soil that is subject to seasonal runoff or that brings gravel, clay and soil. Drought resistant. Can tolerate poor soil.

Time to harvest: Rainy season because trunks ooze gum.

Harvest: The wood is water- and insect-resistant, and produces gum-resign, leaves, flowers, roots, shoots and seedpods. While the seedpods and fresh shoots can be used as a vegetable, the air-dried seeds function as a marginal source of protein for humans in times of duress. Acacia seeds are a good source of food for camel, sheep, goat and cattle. Dried acacia gum powder can be added to almost any dish by mixing or finely sprinkling on the surface.

Attracts friends: Bees and othe rpollinating insects.

Environmental benefits and concerns: Replenishes poor soil, aids in reversing desertification; windbreaker and good boarder trees. Its wood is hard, sturdy, long lasting and resistant to termites and other pests. Acacia has become a serious invasive pest on the continent of Australia.

Storage: Keep fine powdered acacia gum safe in a plastic bag and in a dark and dry place.

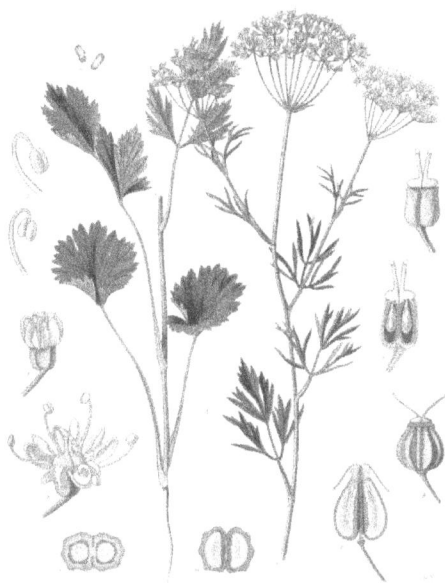

Köhler's Medicinal Plants 1887

Anise

Let life's sensual beauty nurture and protect you from your center to the distant horizons of your mind.

Ancient Greeks and Romans knew this fruit as a delicious aphrodisiac, utilizing it for its digestive and sexually stimulating properties. Similarly, Cubans, traditionally associate anise with Oshun, the goddess of love, sensuality, intimacy, beauty and marriage. The herb's time proven properties echo and honor these associations. Anise (as well as fennel) has been used for thousands of years in traditional healing for its estrogenic properties. In particular, healers have found anise to balance menstrual cycles, enhance a mother's milk secretion, and stimulate libido in women. It has also been discovered that a mother can ease an infant's colic by drinking anise tea while she is breastfeeding. Don't you think the nurturing and loving images conjured

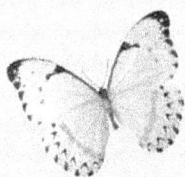

Breathe easy and breathe deep. Remember it can be safe to nurture yourself and another in a manifold of ways upon this magic carpet ride called life. This was true in the beginning and shall be true until the end of time.

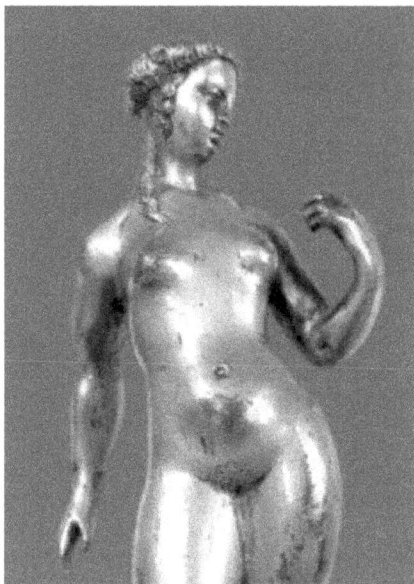

Christohp Weiditz. Venus ca. 1550, gilded bronze. Bode-Museum Berlin

are worthy to be linked to the Goddess of love by whatever name or cultural expression?

Parts used: the ripe fruit

Global summary:

Used to treat: Its therapeutic uses include reducing phlegm, coughs, colds, bronchitis, cramps, and bacterial infections, as well as addressing low immunity, loss of appetite, liver and gall bladder complaints, gastrointestinal problems and possibly hypochondria and panic attacks.

Used a a(n): Expectorant, antispasmodic, antibacterial, estrogen receptor modulator properties, promotes regular menstruation, supports healthy bones, mood elevator, anti-ulcer, carminative (reduces gas), breath freshener, bronchodilator, insect repellent and antifungal.

India:

Anise seed is used as a mouth freshener.

Summary medicinal properties supported by scientific studies:

Anise protects against gastric ulcers, gastro-intestinal difficulties (gas, cramps, bloating), and halitosis (bad breath); used as an antibacterial, expectorant, bronchodilator, anti-spasmotic, mosquito repellant, antifungal (candida); and used for its estrogen receptor modulator-like properties that produce bone-cell formation without causing breast and cervical cancer cell proliferation.

Brazil:

A University of São Paulo study justified the use of anise as an antispasmotic agent.[1] Scientists noted the Brazilian curandeiros' age-old herbal medicinal practices in which anise cured digestive difficulties resulting from gas, overeating, cramps and nervous stomach.

Croatia - Zagreb:

The University of Zagreb[2] tested the effectiveness of anise's fluid extracts and essential oils against several strains of candida in laboratory Petri dishes. Both tested effective for inhibiting fungal growth, although the essential oils proved to contain stronger antifungal properties.

Cuba:

Doctors find the fruit (fresh or dried) effective as an antibacterial and expectorant. It is used to treat coughs and sore throats as well as general low immunity. This Caribbean nation also employs anise's properties for poor digestion, flatulence, hypochondria and panic attacks.

Greece - Athens:
Greek herbalists have used anise and fennel to promote menstruation, increase breast milk production, facilitate birth and enhance libido. University of Athens' scientists have taken a closer look at anise in the context of finding a safe alternative to estrogen replacement therapies in preventing osteoporosis. Anise exhibited estrogen receptor modulator-like properties that produce bone-cell formation without causing breast and cervical cancer cells to proliferate.[3]

Iran - Mashhad:
Iranian scientists discovered a possible mechanism that explains why many traditional healers have been using anise extracts and oils in the treatment of certain respiratory ailments. Anise extracts and essential oils possess bronchodilatory (opens the upper airways) qualities derived from possible antihistamine-like properties.[4] This makes anise oil (or extract) a possible natural allergy treatment or relaxant for upper airway constrictions.

Pakistan - Karachi:
The Indian use of aniseed as a mouth freshener earned scientific merit from a Karachi University study. Scientists describe the oral antibacterial properties against a wide variety of bacteria taken from more than 200 human saliva samples.[5]

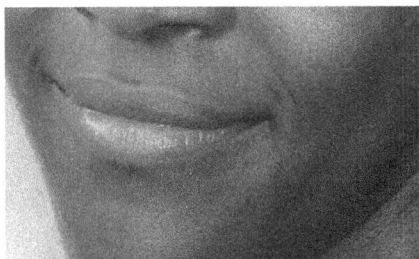

Saudi Arabia - Riyadh:
Since ancient times anise has been used safely in Unani medical tradition, made famous over a 1000 years ago by Hakim Ibn Sina aka Aviciena, to prevent and treat stomach ulcers and other gastro-intestinal complaints. A 2007 King Saud University study confirmed the anti-ulcer properties of a water-based anise solution.[6] The anise solutions, fed to rats at doses of 250mg/kg and 500mg/kg, were noted to provide significant protection against cell-killing agents.

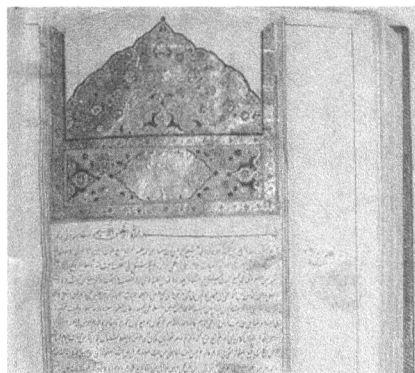

**Ibn Sina. Canon of Medicine ca. 1315.
Courtesy: U.S. National Library of Medicine**

Turkey - Antalya:
Scientists from the Akdeniz University looked at the value of anise seeds' essential oils as a mosquito repellent. A study determined the oils possessed the ability to repel and protect from mosquito bites.[7]

German Commission E:
Approved as an expectorant, antispasmodic agent and antibacterial.

Preparation:
An infusion is prepared by pouring 1/2 liter of boiling water over two to three grams of the dried or fresh fruit. Allow

the herb to sit for 5-7 minutes and drink throughout the day until the infusion is finished.

As a mouth freshener take a few anise seeds and chew them after eating or as needed.

Warning:

There are no known side effects noted with this dosage.

Possible interaction with drugs:

Currently no data is available indicating possible drug interactions.

Amharic: Insilal
Dutch: Anijs
French: Anis cultivé
German: Anis
Hebrew: Anis
Hindi: Saunf
Homeopathic: Illicium (Anis.)
Italian: Anice verde, Anice volgare
Korean: Anisu
Latin: Pimpinela anisum
Russian: Anis
Sanskrit: Shatapushpa
Spanish: Anis

1 Tirapelli CR, de Andrade CR, Cassano AO, De Souza FA, Ambrosio SR, da Costa FB, de Oliveira AM. *Antispasmodic and relaxant effects of the hidroalcoholic extract of Pimpinella anisum (Apiaceae) on rat anococcygeus smooth muscle.* Departamento de Enfermagem Psiquiátrica e Ciências Humanas, Escola de Enfermagem de Ribeirão Preto, Ribeirão Preto, Universidade de São Paulo, Ribeirão Preto, Brazil. J Ethnopharmacol. 2007 Mar 1;110(1):23-9.

2 Kosalec I, Pepeljnjak S, Kustrak D. *Antifungal activity of fluid extract and essential oil from anise fruits (Pimpinella anisum L., Apiaceae).* Department of Microbiology Faculty of Pharmacy and Biochemistry, University of Zagreb, Zagreb, Croatia. Acta Pharm. 2005 Dec;55(4):377-85.

3 Kassi E, Papoutsi Z, Fokialakis N, Messari I, Mitakou S, Moutsatsou P. *Greek plant extracts exhibit selective estrogen receptor modulator (SERM)-like properties.* Department of Biological Chemistry, Medical School, University of Athens, 115 27 Athens, Greece. J Agric Food Chem. 2004 Nov 17;52(23):6956-61.

4 Boskabady MH, Ramazani-Assari M. *Relaxant effect of Pimpinella anisum on isolated guinea pig tracheal chains and its possible mechanism(s).* Department of Physiology, Ghaem Medical Centre, Mashhad University of Medical Sciences, 91735, Mashhad, Iran. J Ethnopharmacol. 2001 Jan;74(1):83-8.

5 Chaudhry NM, Tariq P. *Bactericidal activity of black pepper, bay leaf, aniseed and coriander against oral isolates.* Department of Microbiology, University of Karachi, Karachi-75270, Pakistan. Pak J Pharm Sci. 2006 Jul;19(3):214-8.

6 Al Mofleh IA, Alhaider AA, Mossa JS, Al-Soohaibani MO, Rafatullah S. *Aqueous suspension of anise "Pimpinella anisum" protects rats against chemically induced gastric ulcers.* Department of Medicine, College of Medicine, King Saud University, PO Box 2925 (59), Riyadh 11461, Saudi Arabia. World J Gastroenterol. 2007 Feb 21;13(7):1112-8.

7 Erler F, Ulug I, Yalcinkaya B. *Repellent activity of five essential oils against Culex pipiens.* Akdeniz University, Faculty of Agriculture, Plant Protection Department, 07070 Antalya, Turkey. Fitoterapia. 2006 Dec;77(7-8):491-4.

Growth: Anise is an annual plant that can reach 3-feet hight.

Native to: Mediterranean; but also found around the globe where the climate allows.

How to grow anise: Anise is easy to grow and is best grown from seeds but does not like to be transplanted; so plant where you want it to stay. Sow directly into the garden, after the last frost has passed, in full sun, about ½ inch deep and in rows that are 3-feet apart to avoid crowding. Keep moist until established, and water regularly.

Time to seed: Early spring.

Sun: Full sun.

Zone: 6 – 10.

Soil: Loose, normal but well drained soil.

Time until harvest: About 3-4 months.

Harvest: When you notice that the flowers become heavy with seed-growth they will begin to lean and the petals will die. Take this as your cue. Cut the flowers at this stage and spread them out, one layer deep, on a dry surface and let them finish drying in the sun. Once completely dry, rub the flowers and seeds between your fingers or your hands to separate the seeds, blow gently to separate seeds and flower or use a sieve. Keep the seeds in a dry and dark glass container.

Attracts friends: Butterflies, bees, parasite-eating wasps.

Environmental benefits: Attracts beneficial insects for organic pest control. Adds fragrance and flowers.

Storage: Keep seeds in dry and dark container.

Worlds of Healing

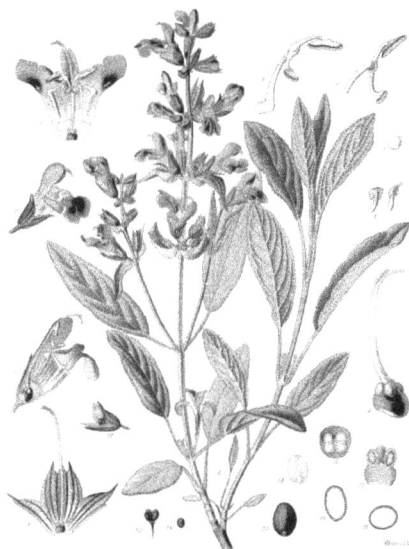

Köhler's Medicinal Plants 1887

Basil

There is a
place in you
where all is
well.

Basil has been a companion of human culinary endeavors for over 4000 years, especially in Asia, Africa and India where it has been a very common addition to food, traditional medicine and spiritual practices. Today, Thailand, Vietnam, Morocco, Cambodia, Laos, Italy and Pakistan find it indispensable.

While there are many different variations of basil this particular exploration focuses on the most commonly found and known type called ocimum basilicum. Its white flowers, hairy stems and deeply green colored leaves are home to a warm, rich, spicy, sweet flavor with a hint of black pepper, clove and mint. A slight rub to a leaf will release its intense scent and envelop your senses.

Parts used: Dried or fresh leaves.

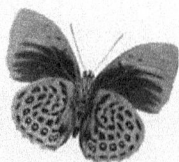

Rub my leaves and I will enter a direct door into your mind. If you let me, I can linger and help you digest stubborn and lingering emotions, assist you in absorbing their remaining treasures with ease. I can help restore your sense of strength and hope. On my scent travels a quiet reminder, to all of those who are willing to listen, there is a place in you where all is well.

Global summary:

Used to treat: dyspepsia (digestive cramps, nausea and vomiting, constipation, flatulence, bloating, colic) high blood pressure, water retention, poor circulation, restlessness, headaches, anxiety, colds, flus, periodic fevers, low energy, exhaustion and loss of appetite.

Used as a(n): antispasmodic, antimicrobial, sedative, diuretic, tonic, appetite and digestive stimulant.

Germany (Hildegard von Bingen):

The famous abbess and healer, offers her millennium old recipe of basil wine, for the treatment of 'Tertian' and 'Quartan' fevers - most likely malaria based fever states. You will need one liter of wine (white), three tablespoons of honey, and a bundle of fresh basil. Bring the wine to a boil and add the basil. Let it simmer for five minutes and pour the content through a sieve. Add the honey. Hildegard von Bingen suggested taking several small glasses throughout the day when the fever was present.

Summary medicinal uses and properties supported by scientific studies:

Antimicrobial (giardia), dyspepsia, high blood pressure (diuretic), potentially effective against cholera toxin induced diarrhea, anti-viral activity against herpes virus I and II, adenoviruses, hepatitis B virus and the RNA viruses (coxsackievirus B1 and enterovirus 71), anti-bacterial (middle ear infection) and anti-inflammatory.

Brazil - Rio de Janeiro:

The essential oil of basil, used in a mouse model, proved an effective agent in the destruction of the common parasite, giardia.[1]

Cuba's clinical uses:

An infusion of basil tea relieves symptoms of abdominal discomfort due to gas. As a diuretic, it treats high blood pressure.

German Commission E:

In 1992, the commission gave basil a negative rating, when a benefit-risk analysis revealed insufficient data for recommending treatment. However, the European Agency for the Evaluation of Medicinal Products wrote in its position 2004 paper on herbal products containing estragole that the dose needed to produce a carcinogenic result would most likely be much higher than at the recommended therapeutic or food based dosages.[2]

Amharic: Besobila
Dutch: Basilicum
French: Basilic
German: Basilikum
Hebrew: Bazilikum
Hindi: Barbar
Homeopathic: Ocimum basilicum
(Oci-b.)
Italian: Basilico
Korean: Basil
Latin: Ocimum basilicum
Russian: Bazilik
Sanskrit: Tulasi
Spanish: Albahaca
Swahili: Mrihani

Iceland - Reykjavik:

Essential oil of basil or some of its isolated components relieved otitis media (middle ear infection) in a rat-based placebo control study when placed topically into the infected ear canals of the rodents.[3]

India - New Delhi:

This albino mice study investigated basil, used extensively in Ayurvedic medicine, and discovered that dosages between 200mg/kg and 400mg/kg of a mixed alcohol/water (80:20) based extract had significant positive impact on anti-oxidant modulation mechanisms. The basil thwarted chemical attempts to produce stomach cancer in the rodents.[4] While conditions, dosages and conclusions of most animal studies cannot be directly translated into a meaningful treatment for humans, the longstanding use of basil in traditional medicine from around the world offers interesting preventative and possible treatment options.

In another rodent study, basil demonstrated strong anti-inflammatory properties affecting the skin surfaces and lining of the intestines.[5]

Mexico:

Scientists tested various botanical extracts' effectiveness in treating diarrhea in a model using rodents. They determined that the water-based extract of basil was highly effective against cholera toxin-induced intestinal secretions.[6]

Morocco - Oujda:

This study looked at basil, a commonly used culinary herb and therapeutic agent of traditional healers in Morocco, with regards to its anti-oxidant properties, and its possible role in reducing cholesterol.[7]

Taiwan - Kaohsiung:

Basil has been used in Traditional Chinese Medicine for thousands of years. Now researchers from the island have taken a closer look at the possible antiviral properties of basil extract and several of basil's specific compounds against DNA viruses, herpes virus, ad-

enoviruses, hepatitis B virus and the RNA viruses (coxsackievirus B1 and enterovirus 71). The results showed that ": ...crude aqueous and ethanolic extracts of basil (ocimum basilicum) and selected purified components, namely apigenin, linalool and ursolic acid, exhibit a broad spectrum of antiviral activity. Of these compounds, ursolic acid showed the strongest activity against HSV-1 ... whereas apigenin showed the highest activity against HSV-2..."[8]

Thailand - Pathumtani:

Basil is a cornerstone in Thai cooking and common in Traditional Thai Medicine. Considered a sacred form of healing, Thai monks have been the unbroken link between the origin of Thai healing to the practices of today. Massage, prayer, spiritual intervention and the use of nutrition and herbs are used to bring about health and healing. Now biotechnologists have confirmed the promising and time-proven antibacterial properties of basil.[9] But, is it the herb alone?

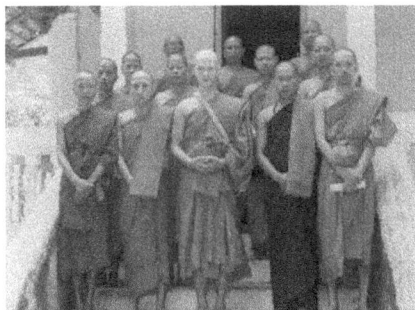

Buddhist monks. Chiang Mai, Thailand. 1981

PREPARATIONS:

Cuba: Pour a liter of boiling water over fifteen grams (half ounce) of dried basil leaves. Let sit for ten to fifteen minutes and then drink six ounces two to three times a day. If using fresh leaves, use thirty grams (about an ounce) with the same preparation.

For flatulence (gas) and abdominal bloating: 150ml of boiling water over two to three grams of the dried herb (one teaspoon is about one and a half grams). The herb sits for about ten to fifteen minutes, is strained, and two to four cups are taken daily in between meals.

Warning:

The essential oil of basil, among many other spices and herbs, contains estragole, which has been found to be carcinogenic in rodent models.[10] Until more information on dose and duration in humans is available it would be prudent not to use basil during pregnancy, while breast-feeding or for infants and young children. However, basil has been part of the human diet for thousands of years with no known side effects from short-term use or in food based dosages.

Possible interaction with drugs:

Currently no data is available indicating possible drug interactions.

1 de Almeida I, Alviano DS, Vieira DP, Alves PB, Blank AF, Lopes AH, Alviano CS, Rosa Mdo S. *Antigiardial activity of Ocimum basilicum essential oil.* Instituto de Microbiologia Prof. Paulo de Góes, Centro de Ciências da Saúde, Universidade Federal do Rio de Janeiro, Rio de Janeiro, RJ, 219491-590, Brazil. Parasitol Res. 2007 Jul;101(2):443-52.

2 The European Agency for the Evaluation of Medicinal Products. *Final Position Paper on the use of Herbal Medicinal Products Containing Estragole.* London. March 3, 2004.

3 Kristinsson KG, Magnusdottir AB, Petersen H, Hermansson A. *Effective treatment of experimental acute otitis media by application of volatile fluids into the ear canal.* Department of Clinical Microbiology, Landspitali University Hospital, Reykjavik, Iceland. J Infect Dis. 2005 Jun 1;191(11):1876-80.

4 Dasgupta T, Rao AR, Yadava PK. *Chemomodulatory efficacy of basil leaf (Ocimum basilicum) on drug metabolizing and antioxidant enzymes, and on carcinogen-induced skin and forestomach papillomagenesis.* Cancer Biology and Applied Molecular Biology Laboratories, School of Life Sciences, Jawaharlal Nehru University, New Delhi, India. Phytomedicine. 2004 Feb;11(2-3-):139-51.

5 Singh S. *Mechanism of action of antiinflammatory effect of fixed oil of Ocimum basilicum Linn.* College of Pharmacy (University of Delhi), Pushp Vihar, New Delhi, India. Indian J Exp Biol. 1999 Mar;37(3):248-52.

6 Velázquez C, Calzada F, Torres J, González F, Ceballos G. *Antisecretory activity of plants used to treat gastrointestinal disorders in Mexico.* Unidad de Investigación Médica en Farmacología de Productos Naturales, Hospital de Pediatría, 2 degrees Piso, Centro Médico Nacional Siglo XXI, IMSS, Col. Doctores, CP 06725, México DF. J Ethnopharmacol. 2006 Jan 3;103(1):66-70.

7 Amrani S, Harnafi H, Bouanani Nel H, Aziz M, Caid HS, Manfredini S, Besco E, Napolitano M, Bravo E. *Hypolipidaemic activity of aqueous Ocimum basilicum extract in acute hyperlipidaemia induced by triton WR-1339 in rats and its antioxidant property.* Department of Biology, Faculty of Sciences, University Mohamed I, Oujda, Morocco. Phytother Res. 2006 Dec;20(12):1040-5.

8 Chiang LC, Ng LT, Cheng PW, Chiang W, Lin CC. *Antiviral activities of extracts and selected pure constituents of Ocimum basilicum.* Department of Microbiology, Kaohsiung Medical University, Kaohsiung, Taiwan. Clin Exp Pharmacol Physiol. 2005 Oct;32(10):811-6.

9 Wannissorn B, Jarikasem S, Siriwangchai T, Thubthimthed S. *Antibacterial properties of essential oils from Thai medicinal plants.* Department of Biotechnology, Thailand Institute of Scientific and Technological Research, Technopolis, Klong-Luang, Pathumthani 12120, Thailand. Fitoterapia. 2005 Mar;76(2):233-6.

10 The European Agency for the Evaluation of Medicinal Products. *Final Position Paper on the use of Herbal Medicinal Products Containing Estragole.* London. March 3, 2004.

Growth: Basil is an annual plant that - depending on species and growing conditions - can vary between 1-foot to 4-feet high.

Native to: India; but is now grown anywhere a sunny and warm climate supports it.

How to grow basil: Basil can easily be grown in the garden or inside in pots. Outside, plant the seed directly into the soil about a ¼ inch deep into trenches. Cover them with good soil and keep them slightly moist until the seeds begin to sprout. Once the plants have a few leaves (3 or 4) you can begin to thin them a bit. Give the plant a little less than a foot of space it will have the space to spread out and develop well, providing you with plenty of leaves to harvest. As soon as flowers appear try to clip them right away to sustain abundant leaf growth.

Time to seed: Plant the seeds in spring after the last frost.

Sun: Full sun.

Zone: 10 – 11.

Soil: Prefers organic, well-drained and rich soil. The plant does not like to be in dry soil.

Time to harvest: You can pick the leaves off the plant as soon as they are mature enough to sustain some picking. Start at the top and pick leaves from several plants so as to spread the potential stress damage and reduce the recovery and re-growth rate.

Harvest: Leaves can be harvested year-round and used in cooking, salads or for medicinal purposes. Frequent picking starting on top encourages more growth, especially when supplied with organic soil support.

Attracts friends: Bees and butterflies.

Environmental benefits: Basil has been reported to repel flies, mosquitoes, aphids, whiteflies and hornworms (a common pest for tomatoes).

Food: Use basil in a thousand dishes and salads.

Storage: Best used fresh but can be dried on a clean cloth in the sun and stored in a dry and dark container.

World of Healing

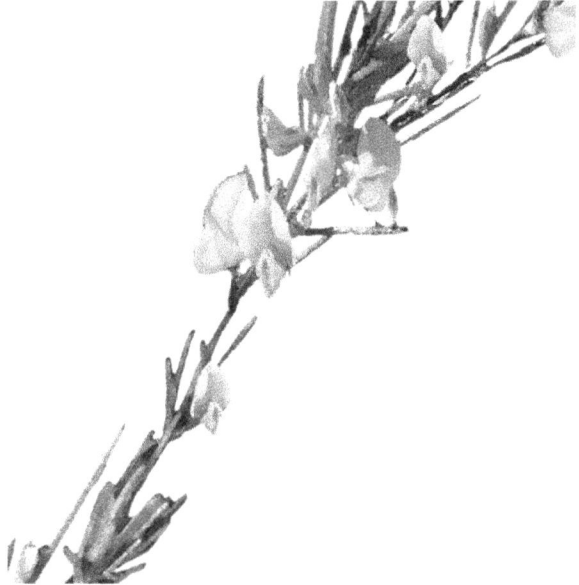

Aspalathus linearis

Bush Tea

'The World is Your Friend' is at once relaxing and functions as a great protective devise.

The forces of ancient winds and the occasional winter rains have sculpted Cederberg Mountain's giant sandstone boulders into bizarre red, yellow, brown and rusty looking shapes. But, these caves and overhangs carved by elemental forces have also been decorated for thousands of years by the Ju'hoansi - or the first people, as the Bushmen call themselves. Bush tea, made from an unassuming plant that reaches about hip high, is caffeine free and apparently unique to the specific Cederberg region of the Western Cape in South Africa. The mountains are situated inland about 250 km north of Cape Town.

To most people, with the exception of the Ju'hoansi, Bush tea remains a relatively new addition to the plethora of therapeutic plants. Today Bush tea is grown as

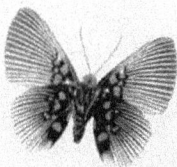

I can help protect you against the stresses of the world but most importantly I can help to nurture and relax. Perhaps you can remember the world is your friend and with that no more protection is needed.

a crop around the South African city of Wuppertal. While not a traditional spice by any means, bush tea, with its deep red coloration in the cup, tastes gentle, sweet, a little woody and makes a great liquid addition to working with spices towards health and healing.

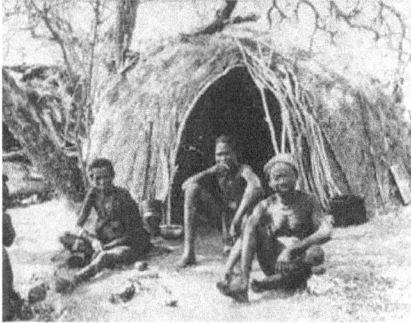

San Tribe in Namibia. Photo by O. Neumeister ca. 1900. Courtesy: Deutsche Kolonialgesell-schaft in der Stadt- und Universitätsbiblio-thek, Frankfurt am Main

Parts used: the ripe fruit

Global summary:
Used to treat: colds, cough and phlegm, nervousness, insomnia, liver problems, poor nutritional conditions, protection against stress factors such as excessive UV light (sun exposure), allergic reactions on the skin and upper airways.
Used a a(n): potent antioxidants, electrolyte replenisher, Bush tea is naturally caffeine-free; acts as a bronchodilator; contains antispasmodic qualities; lowers blood pressure; protects and nurtures liver tissue (Hepaprotector); protects against certain cancers; functions as a cholesterol balancing agent, sleeping aid and helps with allergies (dermatitis).

Medicinal uses and properties supported by scientific studies:
Bush tea protects against certain cancers such as skin cancers and mutations, hyperactive gastrointestinal problems, respiratory difficulty, and high blood pressure. It nurtures and restores the liver and reduces cholesterol.

Japan - Shizuoka:
The Japanese have explored Bush tea's estrogen-based compounds.[1]

Korea - Daejeon:
Laboratory studies have found DNA protective[2] and antimutagenic properties. Studies on animals have indicated immune-controlling properties.

Pakistan - Karachi:
A recent study from Karachi determined why Bush tea is effective in treating hyperactive gastrointestinal problems[3,] respiratory difficulty and high blood[4] pressure. Bush tea is a bronchodilator, antispasmodic and has blood pressure-lowering properties. It apparently achieves this by Portassium (ATP) channel activation with a selective bronchodilatory effect.

Slovak Republic - Dunaji:
Using an animal study, Eastern European scientists demonstrated further therapeutic effects on liver damage such as cirrhosis[5], and a simultaneous reduction in cholesterol by using the plant.

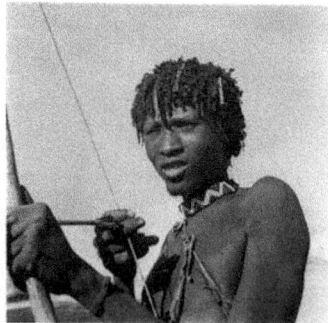

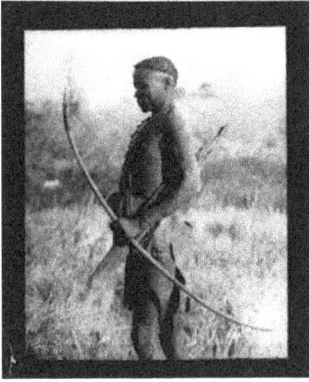

San Tribesman with wild bush 'tea,' Namibia.
Courtesy: Deutsche Kolonialgesellschaft in
der Stadt- und Universitätsbibliothek,
Frankfurt am Main

Africaan: Rooibos
Dutch: Rooibos
French: Rooibos
German: Rotbusch Blüte
Italian: Rooibos
Latin: Aspalanthus linearis
Spanish: Rooibos

South Africa - Tygerberg:

South African researchers who found that topical Bush tea application inhibits skin tumor formation have confirmed the antimutagenic properties of rooibos.[6] Is Bush Tea an 'herbal umbrella' that enables the Ju'hoansi to live and traverse the Kalahari, one of the hottest places on earth?

Botswana:

Bush tea is a very common beverage in Botswana and Namibia. The fictional character of the *Number One Ladies Detective Agency,* Mma-Ramotswe drinks Bush tea throughout her life in the popular novels written by A. McCall Smith.

United States (Boston):

Researchers at the Human Nutrition Research Center on Aging confirmed Bush tea to have antimutagenic abilities, which makes it a potential cancer prevention plant.[7]

Unwanted Effects:

No adverse effects of bush tea consumption as herbal tea have been reported.

PREPARATIONS:

Rooibos tea: use as a beverage throughout the day. Pour one cup of boiling water over one tablespoon of rooibos.

Electrolyte replacement: when sweating a lot on hot days or during athletic exercise.

Soup stock: Prepare a strong rooibos tea and use as a soup stock for your favorite soups.

Skin cream: Use a strong tea and mix a small amount thoroughly with virgin organic coconut oil 1:1 and apply to your skin for soothing relief of dryness or mild sunburn.

WARNING:

None noted.

Possible interaction with drugs:

None noted.

1 Shimamura N, Miyase T, Umehara K, Warashina T, Fujii S. *Phytoestrogens from Aspalathus linearis.* Biol Pharm Bull. School of Pharmaceutical Sciences, University of Shizuoka. 2006 Jun; 29 (6):1271-4.

2 Lee EJ, Jang HD. *Antioxidant activity and protective effect on DNA strand scission of Rooibos tea (Aspalathus linearis).* Department of Food and Nutrition, Hannam University, Daejeon, Korea. Biofactors. 2004; 21(1-4):285-92.

3 Gilani AH, Khan AU, Ghayur MN, Ali SF, Herzig JW. *Antispasmodic effects of Rooibos tea (Aspalathus linearis) are mediated predominantly through K+ -channel activation.* Department of Biological and Biomedical Sciences, Aga Khan

University Medical College, Karachi 74800, Pakistan. Basic Clin Pharmacol Toxicol. 2006 Nov; 99(5):365-73.

4 Khan AU, Gilani AH. *Selective bronchodilatory effect of Rooibos tea (Aspalathus linearis) and its flavonoid, chrysoeriol.* Dept. of Biological and Biomedical Sciences, The Aga Khan University Medical College, Karachi, 74800, Pakistan. Eur J Nutr. 2006 Dec; 45(8):463-9.

5 Ulicna O, Greksak M, Vancova O, Zlatos L, Galbavy S, Bozek P, Nakano M. *Hepatoprotective effect of rooibos tea (Aspalathus linearis) on CCl4-induced liver damage in rats.* Institute of Animal Biochemistry and Genetics, Slovak Academy of Sciences, Moyzesova Str. 61, 900 28 Ivanka pri Dunaji. Slovak Republic. Physiol Res. 2003; 52(4):461-6.

6 Marnewick J, Joubert E, Joseph S, Swanevelder S, Swart P, Gelderblom W. *Inhibition of tumour promotion in mouse skin by extracts of rooibos (Aspalathus linearis) and honeybush (Cyclopia intermedia), unique South African herbal tea*s. PROMEC Unit, Medical Research Council, P.O. Box 19070, Tygerberg 7505, South Africa. Cancer Lett. 2005 Jun 28;224(2):193-202.

7 McKay DL, Blumberg JB. *A review of the bioactivity of south African herbal teas: rooibos (Aspalathus linearis) and honeybush (Cyclopia intermedia).* USDA Human Nutrition Research Center on Aging at Tufts University, 711 Washington St., Boston, MA 02111, USA. Phytother Res. 2006 Aug 23.

Growth: As a wild shrub Bush tea grows up to 6-feet high.

Native to: South Africa's Cedarberg Mountain only.

How to grow bush tea: From seed to mature shrub takes about 2 years. Bush tea only grows in the Cedarberg Mountains of South Africa. The plants make few seeds, which are also very tiny in nature. Plants have been self-propagating in the wild, but some local farmers have been successful at growing them as crops. The seeds are nurtured in shallow soil containing beds until they are about 5-7 inches high and are then planted into the ground around Cedarberg.

Time to seed: The seeds are planted during the South African fall months of February and March; but the plant has so far been determined to only grow in the region from whence it came. Propagation in other countries and regions has not been successful.

Sun: Full sun.

Zone: 8 – 9.

Soil: The plant does well only in the soil and conditions of Cedarberg. The most bioactive tea is from wild crafted plants from areas not clear-cut to promote mono-cultured tea fields. However, as with many other species, wild bush tea and its inherent biodiversity may be endangered from over-use due to worldwide demand, which has risen sharply as local farmers try to meet the global need.

Time to harvest: When the plant has reached a height of 1.5-2 meters or after about 2 years. With the current harvest methods, the shrub - which is not actually a tea plant species but an herb - can produce tea for about 5 years.

Harvest: The needle-like leaves and small stems are harvested in the South African summer November through January. The leaves are dried in the sun and produce a tea more yellow in color with a higher anti-oxidant content. In addition, you can chop the leaves, which allows the fermentation process to take place. The latter technique produces a bright red color and stronger flavor.

Attracts friends: Pollinating insects and birds.

Environmental benefits: Bush tea prevents soil erosion as roots quickly reach deep in search for sparse water.

Food: Caffeine-free beverages and soup stock.

Storage: Bush tea keeps well in a dry, dark and covered container.

Worlds of Healing

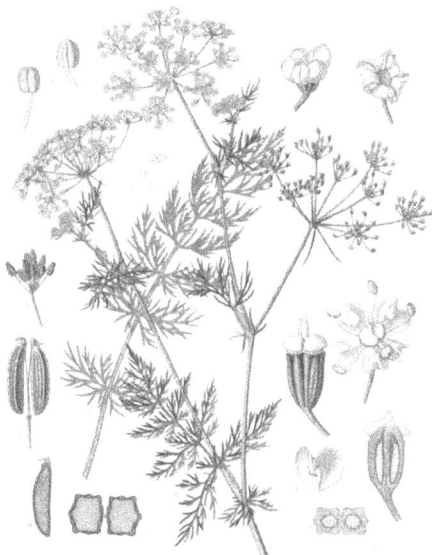

Köhler's Medicinal Plants 1887

Caraway

It is possible
for you to
relax stagnant
ideas and
overwhelming
emotions.

Caraway is another classical addition from the ancient spices and herbs mentioned in age-old Persian records, Africa, Greece, Rome and the Middle Ages. Europeans eat caraway in breads, use the leaves in salads and cook the roots in soups. In the Scandinavian countries, caraway is used in strong liquor called aquavit and as an important ingredient in Sauerkraut. It likes to grow in bright sun and well-drained soil and easily flourishes with plenty of organic fertilizers.

Caraway is often mistaken for cumin, fennel, anise and even licorice. While the scent may be similar, caraway has white flowers; cumin blooms pink; fennel blooms yellow; and licorice looks altogether very different, and instead of using the fruits as with the other three its main part used is the root.

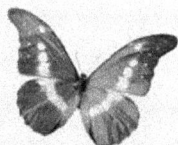

I can help you to fine-tune your digestion, absorption and elimination of your food, may it be physical, mental or emotional. Relax your stagnant ideas and overwhelming emotions. Relax the tightening fear and anxiety in your belly. Relax and let nature take its course. Let life glide through with gentle ease.

Parts used: Fruits and oil.

Global summary:
Used to treat: Various digestive difficulties, including 'nervous stomach' (dyspepsia), colic, gas and bloating, water retention, diabetes, high blood pressure, gastro-intestinal cancer and menstrual cramps.
Used as a(n): Carminative, diuretic, anti-mutagenic, possible colon cancer preventative, hypoglycemic, antimircobial and antispasmodic (reduce cramps - abdominal).

Hildegard von Bingen;
The 11th Century German Abbess and healer extraordinaire used caraway to treat digestive difficulties.

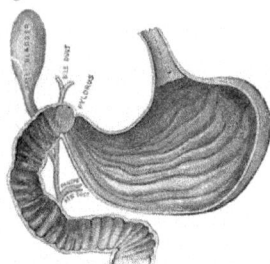

Summary medicinal uses and properties supported by scientific studies:
May prevent mutation, may be useful in the treatment of colon cancer, hypertension, water retention, diabetes and may be helpful in fat metabolism.

German Commission E:
Indicates that sufficient scientific evidence exists to safely use caraway for its antimicrobial and antispasmodic properties.

India - Tamil Nadu:
Caraway has been used in an experimental model on rats to determine if the spice, commonly used in Ayurvedic medicine for gastro-intestinal difficulties, has any impact in the development of chemically induced (with 1,2-dimethylhydrazine) colon cancer. The researchers determined that dietary caraway (at a dose of 60mg/kg) indeed has properties that are able to control lipid peroxidation and anti-oxidant homeostasis, thereby preventing the development of chemically induced colon cancer lesions.[1] Another rodent-based study confirmed these results and further determined that the most optimal dose of the various amounts used in the study was 60mg/kg.[2]

Japan:
In a Department of Molecular Bacteriology study at the Institute of Health Biosciences at the University of Tokushima Graduate School, scientists tested the international awareness placed on caraway as a potential agent to protect against cellular mutations. These scientists believed that a specific compound from caraway called Ogt-O6-methyl-guanine-DNA methyltransferase might be responsible in the antimutagenic activity of caraway.[3]

Morocco - Fez:
North African traditional healers use caraway as a diuretic when water retention, passing urine and, in some cases, high blood pressure need attention. Through an animal study, these Moroccan scientists have now determined that caraway does have strong diuretic properties,[4] which apparently work similarly to the commonly used anti-hypertensive pharmacological drugs Lasix and Hydrochlorthiazide (HCTZ).

What is it about caraway that can bring about water homeostasis and the deeper meaning lying therein?

Morocco - Errachidia:

Another rat-based study from Errachidia looked at the role of caraway (aqueous extract) on fat metabolism, finding that caraway has a significant lipid lowering ability.[5]

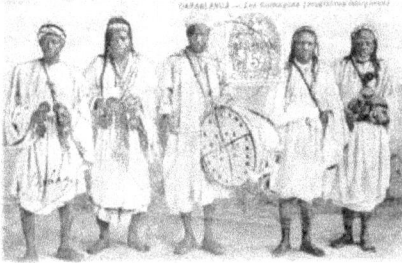

Gnawas, Musicians and traditional healers all at once. Morocco ca. 1920. Courtesy: FayssalF

Morocco - Errachidia:

Errachidia scientists determined from another animal-based study that caraway has the apparent ability to lower blood sugar levels without increasing the body's production of insulin.[6]

PREPARATIONS:

Put a teaspoon of caraway seeds into a cup and pour hot water – let it soak for about five minutes, cool down until comfortable to drink. Consume three times daily with meals.

An average daily dry dose consists of approximately 2-6gm of seeds.

Unwanted Effects: None known.

WARNING:

Like with any water pill, when taking caraway as a diuretic it is possible to lose important minerals, such as potassium, which may lead to cramps and other symptoms.

Possible interaction with drugs:
None noted.

1 Kamaleeswari M, Nalini N. *Dose-response efficacy of caraway (Carum carvi L.) on tissue lipid peroxidation and antioxidant profile in rat colon carcinogenesis.* Department of Biochemistry, Annamalai University, Annamalainagar, 608 002, Tamilnadu, India. J Pharm Pharmacol. 2006 Aug;58(8):1121-30.

2 Deeptha K, Kamaleeswari M, Sengottuvelan M, Nalini N. *Dose dependent inhibitory effect of dietary caraway on 1,2-dimethylhydrazine induced colonic aberrant crypt foci and bacterial enzyme activity in rats.* Department of Biochemistry and Biotechnology, Annamalai University, Annamalainagar 608 002, Tamilnadu, India. Invest New Drugs. 2006 Nov;24(6):479-88.

3 Mazaki M, Kataoka K, Kinouchi T, Vinitketkumnuen U, Yamada M, Nohmi T, Kuwahara T, Akimoto S, Ohnishi Y. *Inhibitory effects of caraway (Carum carvi L.) and its component on N-methyl-N'-nitro-N-nitrosoguanidine-induced mutagenicity.* Department of Molecular Bacteriology, Institute of Health Biosciences, The University of Tokushima Graduate School, Japan. J Med Invest. 2006 Feb;53(1-2):123-33.

Dutch: Wilde komijn
French: Cumin des prés
German: Kümmel
Hebrew: Kimmel
Hindi: Shia jeera
Homeopathic: Carum carvi (Caru.)
Italian: Cumino tedesco
Korean: Karowei
Latin: Carum carvi
Russian: Tmin
Sanskrit: Karavi
Spanish: Carvi
Swahili: Kisibiti

4 Lahlou S, Tahraoui A, Israili Z, Lyoussi B. *Diuretic activity of the aqueous extracts of Carum carvi and Tanacetum vulgare in normal rats.* UFR Physiology-Pharmacology, Laboratory of Animal Physiology, Department of Biology, Fez, Morocco. J Ethnopharmacol. 2007 Apr 4;110(3):458-63.

5 Lemhadri A, Hajji L, Michel JB, Eddouks M. *Cholesterol and triglycerides lowering activities of caraway fruits in normal and streptozoto-*

cin diabetic rats. UFR PNPE B.P. 21, Errachidia 52000, Morocco. J Ethnopharmacol. 2006 Jul 19;106(3):321-6.

6 Eddouks M, Lemhadri A, Michel JB. *Caraway and caper: potential anti-hyperglycaemic plants in diabetic rats.* Laboratory of Endocrinian Physiology, FSTE Boutalamine and Pharmacology, EDDOUKS, UFR PNPE, BP 21, Errachidia 52000, Morocco. J Ethnopharmacol. 2004 Sep;94(1):143-8.

Growth: Caraway is a biennials up to 2-feet high.

Native to: From the region of South-Central Europe to Asia; but nowadays grown anywhere the climate supports it.

How to grow caraway: Caraway is a biennial plant, which means it takes 2 seasons to reach maturity and produce seeds. A little secret: if you want to speed up the process, it sometimes works to plant the seeds in fall and harvest the next summer. However, this is somewhat of a gamble.

Begin planting the seeds in shallow trenches in spring after the first frost has passed; cover them with a thin layer of good soil and keep slightly moist until the first leaves begin to show. Thin the plants so that each plant you want to keep has an umbrella of space measuring about 2 feet to reach its size potential. Keep in mind that caraway does not transplant well. Keep weeds clear from your plants. Caraway can reach up to 2-feet high and has leaves similar to those of carrots.

If you live in areas where you have four marked seasons, mark the spot where you planted the caraway and protect the plant with some mulch during the winter. It will most likely die off but return to complete its growth cycle. Once caraway is established, the plant will self-sow and continuously propagate, sometimes becoming overpowering.

Time to seed: Plant in fall or spring directly into the soil.

Sun: Full sun; but dislikes excessive heat and humidity.

Zone: 3 – 7.

Soil: Organic, fertile soil that drains well but is moisture retentive. The plant can withstand some dry conditions, but once established should be watered about once a week. Add organic compost material once during the season to assure plenty of growth, flowers and seeds.

Time to harvest: Late summer or early fall (usually in September), depending on the dryness of flowers and seeds.

Harvest: Leaves, root and seeds. The leaves can be harvested for your needs as soon as the plant is big enough to sustain the loss of a few. The plant will begin to produce seeds in the second year. The flower of the plant will produce an abundance of caraway seeds. Cut the flowers once they begin to dry and get heavy with seeds. Hang the flower stems upside down covered by a brown paper bag. A fine screen should cover the opening of the bag and catch the seeds as the air drying process is completed. Allow them to dry slowly to preserve the oils. You can also shake the bag to make sure that most seeds dropped down. At the end of the growth cycle you can dig up the roots and use them like a root vegetable similar to that of fennel root or celery.

Attracts friends: Small parasitic wasps, bees, lacewing, hoverflies, pirate bugs and big eyed bugs.

Environmental benefits: Can loosen compacted soil environments and thus support rooting of other plants normally stunned by such conditions.

Food: Leaves are used as garnish in salads soups and many other dishes. The seeds are often used in baking, cheese and soups.

Storage: Caraway seeds with potent oil content keep well for about a year. Keep them in a dry and dark container. They can still be used after that time but it is most likely that most of the plants properties will diminish with time.

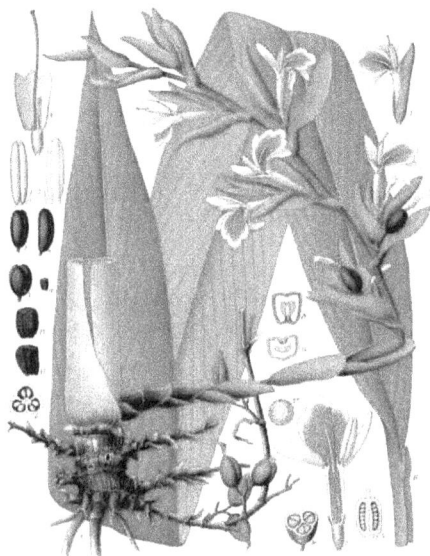

Köhler's Medicinal Plants 1887

Cardamom

There is a place in you where you are bold and strong and beautiful.

Cardamom is one of the world's ancient spices used for thousands of years from the Far East to Mesopotamia to Egypt to Greece Rome and Scandinavia. Viking use of the herb can be found today in popular locally baked goods in Sweden, Norway, Denmark and Finland.

True cardamom, one of two cardamom species, is a very strong smelling perennial plant that grows in the tropical regions of South-East Asia. Reaching up to four meters in height, its intense scent is equally matched by its intense flavor, one employed globally in many culinary delights. The ground seeds contained in the fruit pods, often referred to as "the queen of spices", are crucial for chai tea. Cardamom, valued in many Arabian nations as well as in Ethiopia as a flavoring agent for coffee and teas,

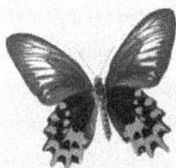

I am strong, I am bold and I am beautiful. I am here to serve and to please and it is my pleasure to remind you of the same qualities in you. If you feel drawn to me, perhaps it is time to re-discover or expand on the boldness, strength and beauty that resides in you.

is mentioned in the Arabian Nights. To this day, many in the Middle East consider it an aphrodisiac. Cineole, a major component of cardamom, is a known stimulant for the central nervous system. Is it the synergy of your pleasure and affinity for this spice that gives rise to elevated energies?

Cardamom spices numerous sweet and savory dishes in India, Bangladesh and Pakistan. The oil of the spice is used in alcoholic beverages, perfumes, cigarettes[1] and sweets. Cardamom is the third most expensive spice in the world, but it takes only a little bit of it to make a big gastronomical impact. It is mostly sold as pods to ensure the freshness and sustained potency of its scent and flavor.

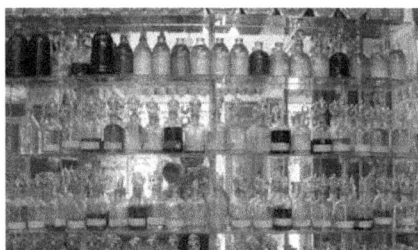

Oils, spices and perfumes. Cairo, Egypt. 2006

Besides its widespread use of culinary enhancements, cardamom also possesses several interesting medicinal properties that have been used as therapeutic agents in Ayurvedic and Unani traditions for a millennia.

Parts used:
Whole dried fruit pods containing the cardamom seeds are sold.

Global summary – medicinal uses:
Used to treat: oral infections, sore throats, upper respiratory infections, tuberculosis, halitosis, eye infections, scorpion and snake bites, skin conditions, liver colic, nausea, vomiting, loss of appetite, and urine retention.

Used as a(n): astringent, stimulant, aphrodisiac, breath freshener, heart stimulant, and as a carminative (aids digestion).

Summary of medicinal uses and properties supported by scientific studies:
May protect against platelet aggregation, lipid peroxidation, and colon cancer. Functions as an anti-spasmodic, anti-inflammatory, anti-viral (genital herpes - HSV-2) and analgesic.

India - Mysore:
Scientists from the city of Mysore, famous for silk, ivory and sandalwood, have discovered that cardamom extract protects platelets[2] from aggregation[3] and lipid peroxidation[4].

India - Kolkata
Nearby, in the city of Kolkata, researchers at the Chittaranjan National Cancer Institute published results of another cardomom study[5]: "These results suggest that aqueous suspensions of cardamom have protective effects on experimentally induced colon carcinogenesis." These findings echo the time-proven Unani and Ayurvedic application of cardamom as

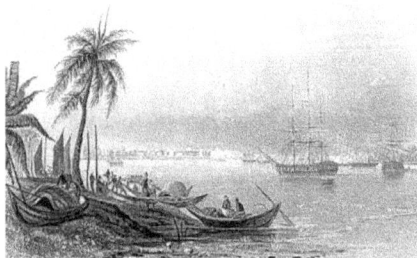

Marine & spice merchants, Calcutta. 1852
Courtesy: Yann

a treatment in certain gastrointestinal diseases.

German Commission E:

Cardamom is an approved drug by the German Commission E in the treatment of dyspepsic complaints (digestive difficulty).

Saudi Arabia - Riyadh:

Researchers at King Saud University uncovered pharmacological abilities of cardamom oil on mammals and determined that cardamom oil exerts its gastrointestinal antispasmodic activity through muscarinic receptor blockage[6]. Moreover, scientists determined that cardamom oil contains anti-inflammatory and analgesic properties.

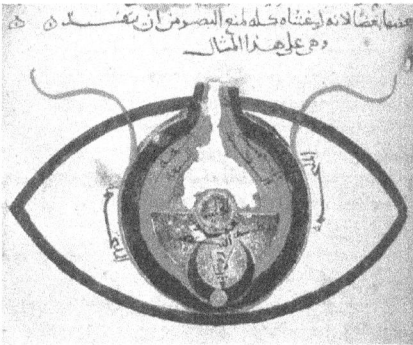

Arabian medical text ca. 12th century. Cairo National Library. Hunain ibn Ishaq. Courtesy: Zereshk

United States - Cincinnati:

At the University of Cincinnati College of Medicine[7] scientists looked at cineole, a major constituent of cardamom, in the context of treating vaginal herpes infections in mice and determined that sufficient evidence exists to warrant more research using this compound as a possibly promising natural treatment modality.

PREPARATIONS:

Commonly used therapeutic dosages of the dry drug are 1.5 gm.

Unwanted Effects:

None known.

WARNING:

Since cardamom stimulates gastric juice production, including those of the gall bladder, it is advisable to exercise caution when using cardamom or any other substance that may aggravate the spasms and pains associated with gallstone conditions.

Possible interaction with drugs:

None known.

1 Cardamom is one of 599 ingredients, which had been a long kept secret, that the five major U.S. cigarette companies supplied to the Dept. of Health and Human Services in 1994. http://www.tobacco.org/Resources/599ingredients.html

2 Suneetha WJ, Krishnakantha TP. *Cardamom extract as inhibitor of human platelet aggregation.* Department of Biochemistry and Nutrition, Central Food Technological Research Institute, Mysore 570 020, India. Phytother Res. 2005 May;19(5):437-40.

3 Platelets are particles in the blood that are essential in the formation of a blood clod – important in closing a wound but may also causing thrombus like in strokes.

4 Lipid peroxidation is a term describing a certain chemical process similar to the rusting of metals. Instead of the metal being oxidized or corroded it is the lipid, the fat that is being oxidized or destroyed.

5 Sengupta A, Ghosh S, Bhattacharjee S. *Dietary cardamom inhibits the formation of azoxymethane-induced aberrant crypt foci in mice and reduces COX-2 and iNOS expression in the colon.* Department of Cancer Chemoprevention, Chittaranjan National Cancer Institute, Kolkata 700026, India. Asian Pac J Cancer Prev. 2005 Apr-Jun;6(2):118-22.

6 al-Zuhair H, el-Sayeh B, Ameen HA, al-Shoora H. *Pharmacological studies of cardamom oil in animals.* Department of Pharmacology, College of Pharmacy, King Saud University, Riyadh, Saudi Arabia. Pharmacol Res. 1996 Jul-Aug;34(1-2):79-82.

7 Bourne KZ, Bourne N, Reising SF, Stanberry LR. *Plant products as topical microbicide candidates: assessment of in vitro and in vivo activity against herpes simplex virus type 2.* Children's Hospital Research Foundation, Department of Pediatrics, University of Cincinnati College of Medicine, OH 45229-3039, USA. Antiviral Res. 1999 Jul;42(3):219-26.

Amharic: Korerima
Dutch: Kardemom
French: Cardamome
German: Kardamom or Hel
Hebrew: Hel
Hindi: Ela(i)chi
Homeopathic: Elletaria cardamomum
                (Elet-c.)
Italian: Cardamomo
Korean: Kadamom
Latin: Elletaria cardamomum
Russian: Kardamon
Sanskrit: Eli
Spanish: Cardamomo

Growth: Cardamom is a perennial up to 4-meters high.

Native to: Tropical Southeast Asia; also grows anywhere else with similar climates.

How to grow cardamom: Cardamom is grown in wild or cultivated gardens in tropical Southeast Asia and is usually propagated by rhizome division. However, cardamom can be grown from fresh, organic, non-irradiated or otherwise treated seeds. The hard seed sprouts more easily if given a signal to initiate growth. A good signal is a cut (not into the core), smoke, hot water or a file/sandpaper scratch Place indoor in pots with rich moist soil to facilitate growth.

Time to seed: Organic environments foster self-propagation for the plant. Cardamom spreads across the forest floor, reaching out a maximum span of 16 feet. The surrounding trees are trimmed and vines and weeds are prevented from overgrowing the plant.

Sun: Needs filtered shade.

Zone: 10 – 11.

Soil: Continuously moist but not muddy.

Harvest: Fall.

Attracts friends: Pollinating bees and hummingbirds.

Environmental benefits: Conserves soil and water, maintains mountain watersheds; good storage of atmospheric carbon; intense and pleasant scent. Gardens can be maintained in the forest without destroying the forest ecology. Large trees are left standing to provide the needed shade. Provides partial and sustainable income for local families who in turn participate in protecting the forest and its biodiversity.

Food: Many foods around the world utilize the seeds' oils and spice.

Storage: Cardamom seeds are best stored left in their pods. Put the pods in a covered glass container and the seeds shoul retain its flavor and properties for many years to come. Powdered cardamom does not store well or long.

Worlds of Healing

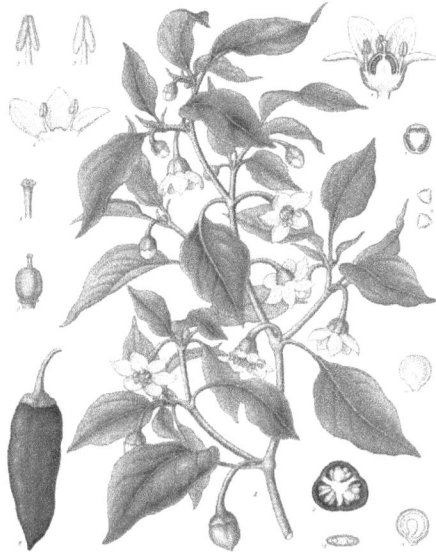

Köhler's Medicinal Plants 1887

Cayenne

Release old
pains and
standing
angers and
you too can
emerge anew
like the
phoenix.

Cayenne peppers are mostly bushy perennials that, according to the current consensus, were originally cultivated by indigenous people of Central and South America. Nowadays, cayenne peppers are grown all over the world where the climate allows. All of this plant's many varieties can be grown easily in most gardens from the tropics to tempered regions. Taste, color, shape and degree of spiciness of any one plant of this family depends greatly on where and how it is grown.

For thousands of years, cayenne has been used for spice and therapeutic needs. Recently, as a defensive weapon, it gained popularity as the stinging ingredient in "pepper sprays". However, the punishing aspect of cayenne is by no means new. Cayenne use can be traced to discouraging thumb

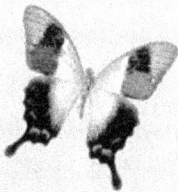

I am red, I am hot, I am fire. I will make you sweat. My heat can awaken and help you release old pains and angers. It can assist you in burning away irritation and annoyance to emerge peaceful and in balance with your self. Practice discernment with me and I will help you balance with nature. I stimulate and invigorate, but take too much and you will get burned.

sucking in children and weaning babies with cayenne-covered nipples. Additionally, it's been utilized to dispel pests and serve in some forms of torture. The range of cayenne's uses - spice, cosmetics, aphrodisiac, therapy, as a weapon - reveals only part of its versatility, making it some what of a wonder drug.

Parts used: Dried, fresh fruit and flower

Global summary:
Used to treat: inflammation in the joints, arthritis, rheumatism, lumbago, neuralgia, neuropathies, muscle spasms and pains, fevers, sore throat (as a gargle), colds, gum infections, arteriosclerosis, malaria fever.
Used as a(n): anti-inflammatory, anti-hemorrhoidal, blood cleanser, malaria prevention, a tonic, and to reduce high cholesterol.

Indigenous tribes have used topical applications to re-grow hair-loss in males and as a beauty enhancement bath. Poultices have been applied to external tumors and employed to draw out snake and insect poison. Internally, some

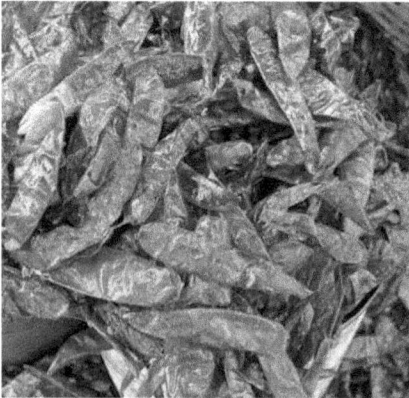

Cayenne pepper. Makola Market, Accra 2008.

tribes use cayenne as a malaria prevention and a decongestant.

In fever, cayenne has been used as a diaphoretic (produces sweating - cayenne is hot on mucus membranes but reduces pains on other skin tissue). Taken as a tonic to clean the blood, it reduces the craving for alcohol and prevents arteriosclerosis, arthritis flare-ups, stroke and heart disease.

Cayenne is used as a stimulant, and is

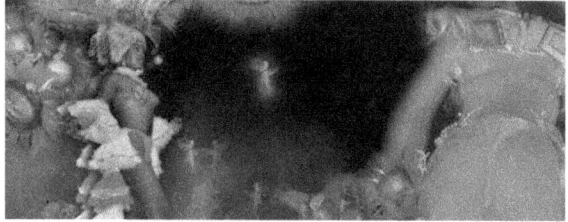

valued as an aphrodisiac worldwide. Creams containing capsaicin (one of the main compounds in cayenne) are sold to treat psoriasis or arthritis pains. Simple, inexpensive homemade creams with fresh and potent peppers are more effective.

Can one plant really treat so many different medical conditions? Can cayenne rid tumors and some forms of cancer? Does cayenne prevent or cure stomach ulcers? And, what of these claims worldwide:

Jamaica: it prevents malaria.
Columbia: it neutralizes poisonous snake venom.
Cuba: provides arthritis relief.
Thailand: treats diabetes.

Besides the case studies from all over the world, other scientific evidence provides further evidence of these claims.

Summary medicinal uses and properties supported by scientific studies:
Used to: enhance circulation where applied, balance fat and sugar metabolism,

protect the stomach lining, can produce significant prostate cancer apoptosis (death), analgesic (for chronic pains such as arthritis, lumbago, rheumatism), anti-venom, anti-tumor, a treatment for shingles, anti-fungal (inc. C. albicans) and anti-bacterial.

Canada - Toronto:
In a meta-analysis of studies, University of Toronto doctors determined that cayenne cream used as a topical ointment was able to better treat the symptoms of chronic back pain than a placebo.[1]

Colombia - Medellin:
Dozens of herbal extracts have been found to either completely or moderately neutralize snake poison when injected together with the poisonous pit viper (Bothrops atrox) venom. Cayenne has a moderately neutralizing effect.[2] Columbian healers showed scientists how cayenne acts as an extract when used in traditional medicine as a poultice, drawing out the poison from snake and scorpion bites.

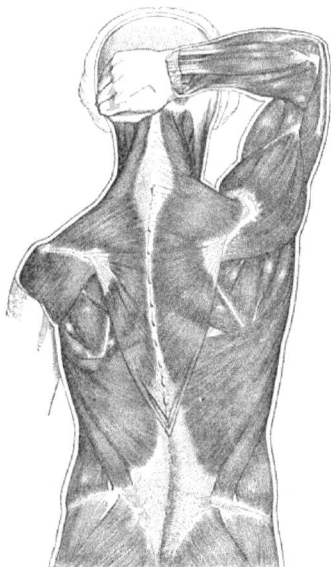

Cuba's clinical uses:
Cayenne stimulates peripheral circulation. In Cuba, a topical tincture and cream produces circulatory benefits when used to treat specific chronic aches and pains as in lumbago, arthritis and rheumatism.

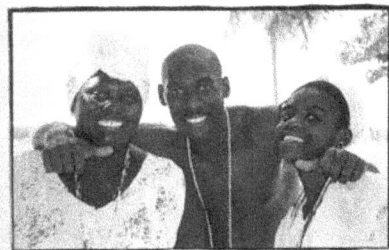

Santeristas Trinidad, Cuba.
Courtesy: Oreet Rees

Cuba's traditional uses:
Used to prevent microbial infections transmitted by lice, scabies and mosquitoes, cayenne belongs to Chango, the passionate God of thunder and lightning.

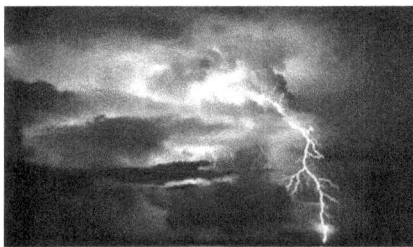

Image courtesy: U.S. National Oceanic and Atmospheric Administration

Germany - Frankfurt:
The fat and sugar balancing effects of cayenne (among other herbs) have been documented at the Johann Wolfgang Goethe University. A present study provides rationale for the use of cayenne in diabetic treatment.[3]

German Commission E:
Approved as an external application for painful muscle spasms. Not to be used for longer than two days on the same region of tissue in order to avoid local skin inflammation.

Singapore:
For years, people have believed that spicy foods such as cayenne caused stomach ulcers. However, a recent study indicates that cayenne pepper actually protects the stomach mucosa.[4] Presently, allopathic medicine believes that most ulcers are caused by a bacterium called helicobacter pylori and/or from the use of anti-inflammatory drugs such as aspirin, acetaminophen, ibuprofen or naproxen.

Spain - Madrid:
After studying cayenne and prostate cancer in the laboratory and in patients, scientists concluded that capsaicin in cayenne "is a promising anti-tumor agent in hormone-refractory prostate cancer, which shows resistance to many chemotherapeutic agents."[5]

Thailand - Bangkok:
Doctors noted an increase in metabolic rates and a slowing down of sugar (glucose) uptake after giving 5gm of fresh cayenne to a group of Thai women.[6] This, in turn, may provide scientists with more reasons why traditional healers world-wide have been using cayenne as a means to treat certain forms of diabetes.

United States - Farmington:
Injecting capsaicin directly into a tumor resulted in the retardation not just of the injected tumor but also of other similar tumors nearby.[7] Although tested in an animal model, scientists know from prior or discoveries that dendrite cells (tree-like extensions of nerve cells) have receptors that when engaged by capsaicin produce significant chemical changes which enhance the body's own immunity.

The FDA approved a cream, under the brand name Zostrix, which contains concentrated capsaicin. The company markets the cream mostly to arthritis sufferers to reduce pain, but also to reduce the pain that often lingers after an attack of shingles (a herpes-caused skin infection). A tube of Zostrix cream usually sells for about fifteen to twenty dollars.

A homemade cayenne pepper cream costs pennies in comparison.

United States - New Orleans:
Scientists, from the 'Big Easy', probably no strangers to wonderfully spicy foods, have determined that an isolated compound made from cayenne is effective in the laboratory against a variety of fungus, including Candida albicans.[8]

United States - Athens:
Ohio University scientists looked at the use of cayenne in Mayan traditional medicine and confirmed its anti-bacterial and anti-fungal properties.[9]

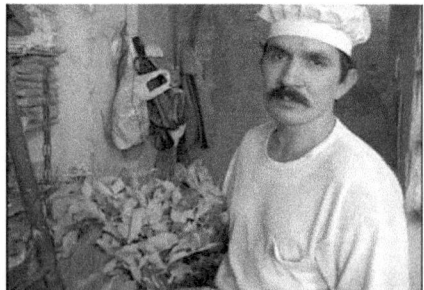

Herbalist. Havana, Cuba

PREPARATIONS:

Cayenne can be used in capsules, creams, lotions, poultices and tinctures. However, Cuban herbalists do not like to use capsules because they believe that the therapeutic chemical reaction starts in the mouth and the experience of tasting it is an extremely important part of the cure. Do oral sensations and tastes play a role in the therapeutic effects of the spice?

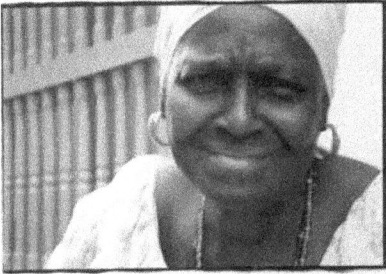

Old Havanna, Cuba

Unwanted Effects:

Skin inflammation. May cause painful burning sensation when in contact with mucus membranes and open wounds.

WARNING:

Cayenne taken in high dosages and/or over a long period of time can cause gastritis and diarrhea. Topically, it can cause skin irritation and blisters. High concentrations have also been known to cause liver and kidney problems. Start slowly and build up a tolerance for maximum beneficial effects.

Possible interaction with drugs:

Anti-inflammatory drugs such as aspirin, acetaminophen, ibuprofen or naproxen can cause stomach ulcers and gastro-intestinal bleeding. Cayenne may protect or diminish the damage of these non-steroidal anti-inflammatory

drugs by protecting the mucus lining inside the stomach.

A study conducted on rats from the South of India determined that a slightly different species of the plant family, capsium annum - chili pepper, when combined with a chemical known to produce colon cancer called 1,2-dimethylhydrazine (DMH) apparently enhanced colon cancer formation.

1 Gagnier JJ, van Tulder MW, Berman B, Bombardier C. *Herbal medicine for low back pain:* a Cochrane review. Institute of Medical Science, Faculty of Medicine, University of Toronto, Toronto, Ontario, Canada. Spine. 2007 Jan 1;32(1):82-92.

2 Otero R, Núñez V, Barona J, Fonnegra R, Jiménez SL, Osorio RG, Saldarriaga M, Díaz A. *Snakebites and ethnobotany in the northwest region of Colombia. Part III: neutralization of the hemorrhagic effect of Bothrops atrox venom.* Programa de Ofidismo, Facultad de Medicina, Universidad de Antioquia, A.A. 1226, Medellín, Colombia. J Ethnopharmacol. 2000 Nov;73(1-2):233-41.

3 Rau O, Wurglics M, Dingermann T, Abdel-Tawab M, Schubert-Zsilavecz M. *Screening of herbal extracts for activation of the human peroxisome proliferator-activated receptor.* Johann Wolfgang Goethe University Frankfurt, Institute of Pharmaceutical Chemistry/ZAFES, Frankfurt/Main, Germany. Pharmazie. 2006 Nov;61(11):952-6.

4 Yeoh KG, Kang JY, Yap I, Guan R, Tan CC, Wee A, Teng CH. *Chili protects against aspirin-induced gastroduodenal mucosal injury in humans.* Department of Medicine, National University Hospital, Singapore. Dig Dis Sci. 1995 Mar;40(3):580-3.

5 Sánchez AM, Sánchez MG, Malagarie-Cazenave S, Olea N, Díaz-Laviada I. *Induction of apoptosis in prostate tumor PC-3 cells and inhibition of xenograft prostate tumor growth by the vanilloid capsaicin.* Department of Biochemistry and Molecular Biology, School of Medicine, University of Alcalá, Alcalá de Henares, Madrid, 28871, Spain. Apoptosis. 2006 Jan;11(1):89-99.

6 Chaiyata P, Puttadechakum S, Komindr S.

Effect of chili pepper (Capsicum frutescens) ingestion on plasma glucose response and metabolic rate in Thai women. Research Center, Ramathibodi Hospital, Mahidol University, Bangkok 10400, Thailand. J Med Assoc Thai. 2003 Sep;86(9):854-60.

7 Beltran J, Ghosh AK, Basu S. *Immunotherapy of tumors with neuroimmune ligand capsaicin.* Center for Immunotherapy of Cancer and Infectious Diseases, University of Connecticut School of Medicine, 263 Farmington Avenue, Farmington, CT 06030-1601, USA. J Immunol. 2007 Mar 1;178(5):3260-4.

8 De Lucca AJ, Bland JM, Vigo CB, Cushion M, Selitrennikoff CP, Peter J, Walsh TJ. *CAY-I, a fungicidal saponin from Capsicum sp. fruit. Southern Regional Research Center,* Agricultural Research Service, US Department of Agriculture, New Orleans, LA 70124, USA. Med Mycol. 2002 Apr;40(2):131-7.

9 Cichewicz RH, Thorpe PA. *The antimicrobial properties of chile peppers (Capsicum species) and their uses in Mayan medicine.* Department of Environmental and Plant Biology, Ohio University, Athens 45701, USA. J Ethnopharmacol. 1996 .

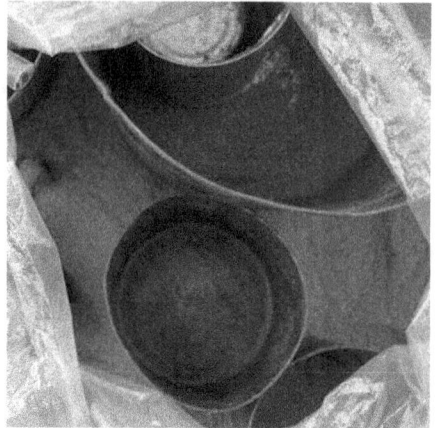

Cayenne. Macola Market, Accra, Ghana

Amharic: Mitmita
Dutch: Paprika
French: Poivre rouge
German: Paprika
Hebrew:Paprika harifa
Hindi: Lal mirch
Homeopathic: Capsicum annum only
            (Caps.)
Italian: Peperoncino, Capsico
Korean: Kochu
Latin: Capsicum frutescens
Russian:Chilli
Sanskrit:Marichiphala Ujjvala
Spanish: Aji picante
Tigrinya: Mitmita

Growth: This cayenne pepper is an annual (e.g. North America) and perennial (e.g. Central and South America), depending on the climate; reaches not quite 2-feet high.

Native to: South America (most likely).

How to grow cayenne: Cayenne peppers are relatively easy to grow. Seeds can be placed straight into the soil or started in seedbeds or pots.

Time to seed: Springtime, once the frost has passed and you are sure the ground will stay warm.

Sun: Outside of their native hot climates the cayenne peppers need full sun. Consider some shade during the peak sun hours to reduce the potential for sun-damage.

Zone: 9 – 11.

Soil: Work the soil with organic compost and prepare by loosening. Use mulch to support even moisture content. Too dry or excessively moist soils will diminish the plant's strength.

Harvest: Late summer or fall. Sizes of cayenne peppers may vary, depending on the species; they usually extend 2-6 inches in length. It takes about 3 months from seed to harvest. Pick the peppers when they transition from green to a full red color and snap off easily. However, it is better to cut the cayenne peppers to reduce the injury rate to the plant. Also, remember to not touch your eyes or other mucus membranes once handling cayenne to avoid burning sensations.

Attracts friends: Flowering plant attracts Bees especially on hot days.

Environmental benefits and concerns: Powdered cayenne pepper, hot pepper spray, tinctures or wax is used by some as an animal or insect deterent. However, it is a relatively violent method to painfully irritate the mucusmembranes in the snouts, noses and eyes of squirrls, deer, gofers, mice, rabbits as well as your own cats and dogs. There are more humane means to perhaps achieve the same goals.

Food: Fresh in salsas or sauces, dried or pickled as seasoning.

Storage: Keep dried whole peppers or powdered pepper in a dry, tight glass jar and in a dark spot to maintain potent taste and properties.

Worlds of Healing

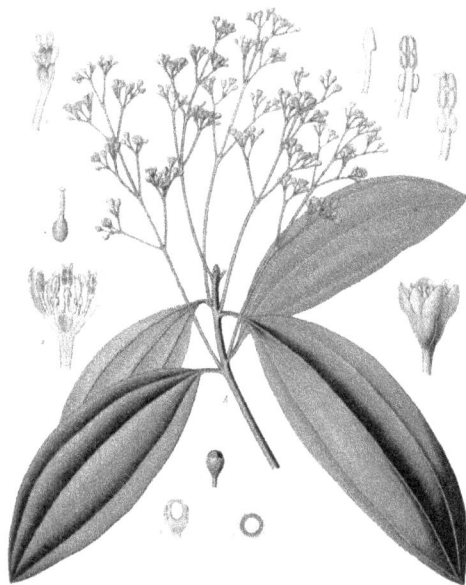

Köhler's Medicinal Plants 1887

Cinnamon

Breathe, you
are alive.

Cinnamon, an evergreen tree native to Sri Lanka and the South of India, reaches heights of 15 meters. The strong unmistakable smell of cinnamon once earned it a highly prized reputation for aphrodisiacal powers.

As a medicine in ancient times, merchants traded cinnamon with the royal courts of early China and Egypt. One finds mention of it in the Old Testament, Exodus 30:23.

Later, empires such as Rome and Greece commonly traded cinnamon as a highly prized commodity. In the Middle Ages, traders from Venice distributed cinnamon throughout Europe to the few with the means able to afford it. Arabian traders kept the origin of the plant secret for many generations telling tales worthy for inclusion in "The Book of One Thousand and One Nights".

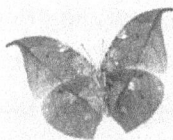

My scent is unmistakable and arouses the senses. Love and passion rides in between the undulating whiffs of my skin. Breathe deep and relax and remember that to enjoy yourself can be as easy as the smelling of my skin.

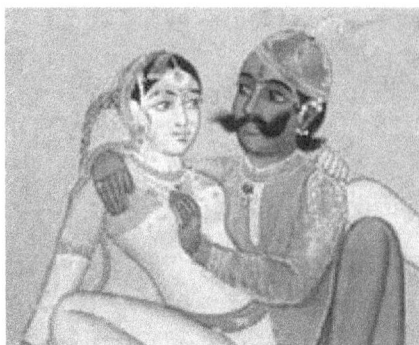

Kama Sutra

It is mentioned in the Kama Sutra. In addition, Grenadian women as well have used cinnamon to attract a lover. It is said that placing a cinnamon stick in your mouth will help to increase the power of seduction while a bath with the herb may facilitate the arousal of intense passions. On the neighboring island of Cuba where the ancient African Gods still rule today cinnamon is an herb that belongs to the goddess Oshun, the Goddess of love.

Ancient myth? Superstition? No, says Neurologist Dr. Alan Hirsch, Director of Chicago's Smell and Taste Treatment and Research Foundation, who found that male sexual stimulation increases when men are exposed to the scent of cinnamon.

Parts used:
Dried flowers and the dried peeled bark of small branches.

Global summary:
Used to treat: Nausea, lack of appetite, low energy, bloating, gas and digestive, abdominal cramps, some forms of sexual dysfunction, hypertension, colds, sore throat, low immunity, psoriasis, bacterial infections, malaria and mild forms of asthma. An Indian home remedy used in the treatment of mild asthma is to take one teaspoon of honey and mix it well with a half a teaspoon of cinnamon powder.

Cuba's traditional uses:
It is used as a syrup to treat gastrointestinal difficulties such as diarrhea and vomiting. Cinnamon is well known in every Cuban city as one of the herbs belonging to Oshun, the goddess of love. Women have used cinnamon since ancient times to attract a lover. It is said that placing a cinnamon stick in your mouth will help to increase the power of seduction, while a bath with the herb arouses intense passions.

Middle East:
Cinnamon oil is known in the Arab world as an oil rub to increase erotic stimulation.

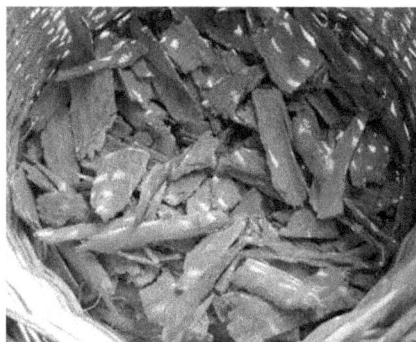

Summary medicinal uses and properties supported by scientific studies:
May improve fat and sugar metabolism; may reduce high blood pressure may work as an antioxidant; includes broad-spectrum antibiotics properties; may enhance sugar and fat metabolism; and, cures mite infestation in animals.

Canada - Calgary & Laval:
Canadian researchers have determined that cinnamon may be a valuable candi-

date for new anti-diabetic medications.[1] A Quebec study has determined cinnamon's effectiveness in the treatment of gastroin-testinal difficulties in traditional cultures wherever it is grown or traded. The Quebec study also found that cinnamon oil increases acidity inside the cells of E. coli, thereby damaging the invading bacteria cell's membrane, causing its death.[2]

China - Hongkong:
Barefoot doctors in rural China use cinnamon sticks to prepare a decoction, which is used in the treatment of: aching joints, male sexual dysfunction, the unusual absence of menstruation, diarrhea, and bed-wetting. A Hong Kong study also suggests that cinnamon possesses broad-spectrum antibiotic properties.[3]

Cuba's clinical uses:
A cinnamon infusion is prescribed to stimulate appetite and the immune system in patients with tendencies toward bacterial and fungal infections.

India - Mysore:
Cinnamon is widely used in Ayurvedic medicine in the treatment of diabetes. Similar to their Canadian colleagues, Tamil Nadu studies indicate that cinnamon contains hypoglycemic and hypolipidemic properties[4] and improves glucose metabolism.[5] Another Indian study in Mysore revealed that a cinnamon fruit powder water extract contains potent antioxidant properties.[6]

Italy - Pisa:
A veterinary study conducted in Italy found that the essential oil of cinnamon was 100% effective in the treatment of mite-infested rabbits.[7]

United States - Chicago:
Neurologist Alan Hirsch, Director of Chicago's Smell and Taste Treatment and Research Foundation, established that male sexual stimulation increases with exposure to the scent of cinnamon. Furthermore, researchers from Washington concluded that cinnamon might also play a beneficial role in lowering high blood pressure.[8]

Commission E:
Approved for the treatment of: "Loss of appetite, dyspeptic complaints such as mild spasms of the gastrointestinal tract, bloating, flatulence."

Preparation:
Crush approximately 2-3gm of the bark into a fine powder and pour a cup of cool water over it and bring to a boil. Let it sit for about ten minutes, cool and drink up to three cups a day.

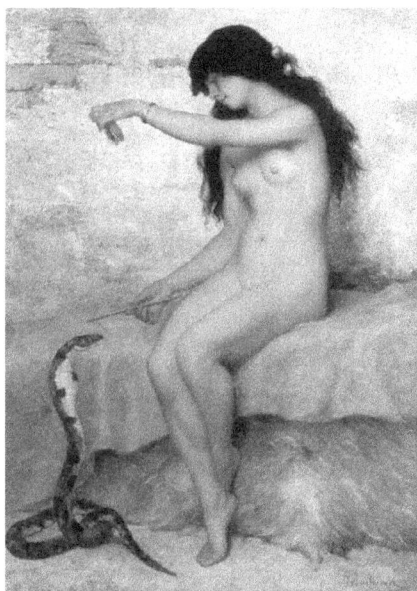

Paul Désiré Trouillebert ca. 1880

WARNING:

Generally, cinnamon is a very safe herb to use but some cases have been reported in which people developed sensitivity to cinnamon. As always be careful with the essential oil.

Possible interaction with drugs:

Currently no data is available indicating possible drug interactions.

Amharic: Kerefa
Dutch: Kaneel
French: Cannelle de Chine
German: Zimt
Hebrew: Kassia
Homeopathic: Cinnamomun
*   (Cinnam.)*
Italian: Cannella della Cina
Korean: Kasia
Latin: Cinnamomum Aromaticum
Russian: Kasia
Spanish: Canela
Twi: Anoatredua

1 Kim W, Khil LY, Clark R, Bok SH, Kim EE, Lee S, Jun HS, Yoon JW. *Naphthalenemethyl ester derivative of dihydroxyhydrocinnamic acid, a component of cinnamon, increases glucose disposal by enhancing translocation of glucose transporter.* Julia McFarlane Diabetes Research Centre and Department of Microbiology and Infectious Diseases, Faculty of Medicine, University of Calgary, Calgary, AB, Canada. Diabetologia. 2006 Oct;49(10):2437-48.

2 Oussalah M, Caillet S, Lacroix M. Mechanism of action of Spanish oregano, *Chinese cinnamon, and savory essential oils against cell membranes and walls of Escherichia coli O157:H7 and Listeria monocytogenes.* Canadian Irradiation Center and Research Laboratory in Sciences Applied to Food,

Institut Nacional de la Recherche Scientifique, Institut Armand-Frappier, Universite du Quebec, 531 Boulevard des Prairies, Laval, Quebec, Canada. J Food Prot. 2006 May;69(5):1046-55.

3 Ooi LS, Li Y, Kam SL, Wang H, Wong EY, Ooi VE. *Antimicrobial activities of cinnamon oil and cinnamaldehyde from the Chinese medicinal herb Cinnamomum cassia Blume.* Department of Biology, The Chinese University of Hong Kong, Shatin, N.T., Hong Kong, People's Republic of China. Am J Chin Med. 2006;34(3):511-22.

4 Subash Babu P, Prabuseenivasan S, Ignacimuthu S. Phytomedicine. *Cinnamaldehyde-A potential antidiabetic agent.* Division of Ethnopharmacology, Entomology Research Institute, Loyola College, Chennai 600 034, Tamil Nadu, India. 2007 Jan;14(1):15-22. Phytomedicine. 2007 Jan;14(1):15-22

5 Kannappan S, Jayaraman T, Rajasekar P, Ravichandran MK, Anuradha CV. *Cinnamon bark extract improves glucose metabolism and lipid profile in the fructose-fed rat.* Department of Biochemistry, Annamalai University, Annamalai Nagar, Tamil Nadu 608002, India. Singapore Med J. 2006 Oct;47(10):858-63.

6 Jayaprakasha GK, Ohnishi-Kameyama M, Ono H, Yoshida M, Jaganmohan Rao L. *Phenolic constituents in the fruits of Cinnamomum zeylanicum and their antioxidant activity.* Central Food Technological Research Institute, Mysore, India. J Agric Food Chem. 2006 Mar 8;54(5):1672-9.

7 Fichi G, Flamini G, Zaralli LJ, Perrucci S. *Efficacy of an essential oil of Cinnamomum zeylanicum against Psoroptes cuniculi.* Dipartimento di Patologia Animale, Profilassi ed Igiene degli Alimenti-Faculty of Veterinary Medicine of Pisa University, Italy. Phytomedicine. 2007 Feb;14(2-3):227-31.

8 Preuss HG, Echard B, Polansky MM, Anderson R. *Whole cinnamon and aqueous extracts ameliorate sucrose-induced blood pressure elevations in spontaneously hypertensive rats.* Department of Physiology, Georgetown University Medical Center, Washington, DC 20057, USA. J Am Coll Nutr. 2006 Apr;25(2):144-50.

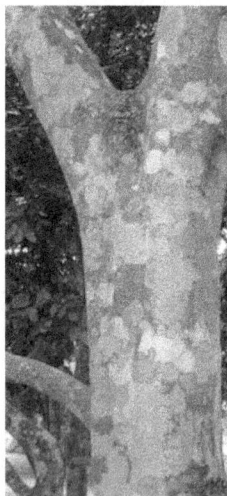

Growth: Cinnamon is a tropical and sub-tropical evergreen tree that grows between 18-30 feet high.

Native to: Cinnamon trees were apparently once indigenous to the island of Sri Lanka-more specifically the Sinharaja rainforest. Nowadays, the tree grows in parts of India, Bangladesh, Indonesia, South-America, Southeast Asia, the Caribbean islands and in parts of tropical Africa (such as Ghana or the islands of Zanzibar and Madagascar).

How to grow cinnamon: Wild cinnamon trees are quite different from farmed cinnamon trees, which are grown for about two to three years until the roots are well established. The tree is then cut down. Dozens of thin shoots will soon spring from the edge of original tree stump. These are harvested every rainy season. Actually, it's the bark that is harvested from these little finger-size shoots. The bark is stripped off and cut into shorter strips and dried. The bark curls as if still trying to clothe the shoot and hardens in place, which is why the sticks look the way they do.

Cinnamon trees do not like to be disturbed once roots have taken place. Grown from seed or cultivated from cutting starts in pots or trays but requires the right environment and care to flourish, especially when outside its native habitat. Although it takes more effort, it is possible to grow cinnamon elsewhere.

Time to seed: Year around in its native habitat.

Sun: Prefers tropical sunshine with partial shade. Can be grown outside the tropics, but can't handle frost very well or prolonged cool periods.

Zone: 9 – 11.

Soil: Deep layers of well drained soil rich in nutrients and frequent rain.

Harvest: The rainy season makes the bark softer which in turn makes it easier to strip the bark from the shoots. Cinnamon is harvested after each rainy season. Strip the bark's outer layer from its shoots, cut them into the desired lengths and dry them in a dark space until they are hard. That's it - at least as far a 'novice' is concerned.

Sri Lanka is the island country with the oldest and undoubtedly most proud tradition of procuring the best cinnamon in the world. Cinnamon growers and cutters are on the top of their game having perfected the complex art and skill of growing, cutting and curing the island's cinnamon that requires seasoned knowledge and experience.

However, a wild cinnamon tree will allow you to take a clipping of a small branch. Grind away at the bark for the cinnamon you need. If you cut from the main trunk, take small pieces only and do not cut across the circumference of the bark or you will kill the tree.

Attracts friends: The spicy, sweet smelling white flowers and bark attract birds and bees.

Environmental benefits: Many cinnamon farms, especially on Sri Lanka, are organic small-time home-growers who make an economically and environmentally sustainable living on a relatively small space.

Food: Cinnamon is used in a great many dishes, savory and sweet alike.

Storage: Cinnamon can last virtually forever if stored in a dry and dark place. However, it may lose its flavor and properties if ground and stored over time. Best to grind the amount you need at the time.

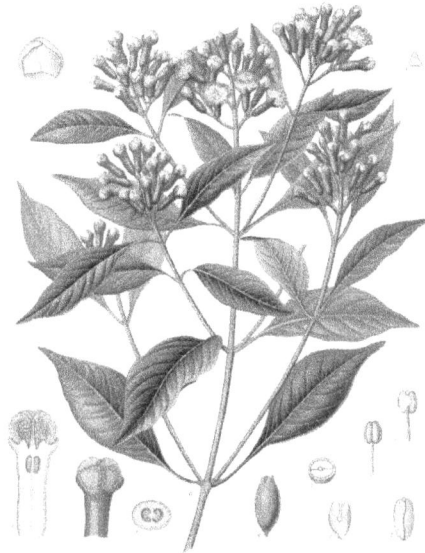

Köhler's Medicinal Plants 1887

Clove

Life is incredibly
and wondrously
intense - enjoy.

The clove, an evergreen tree ranging in height from 30 to 60 feet, bears crimson-colored flowers that are picked and dried to become a spice that has been used worldwide since ancient times.

Clove was traded along the spice routes for thousands of years from China through the Indus Valley, the Middle East to Northern Africa and all the way to Northwestern Europe where it has been appreciated for its intense flavor, taste and scent. While now inexpensive and readily available, a few hundred years ago it was rare in Europe and highly prized. It has been used in medicine as an aphrodisiac, a spice, a cigarette flavor and as a room deodorizer.

While the Indonesian islands produce most of the world's clove, other major regions include Sri Lanka, India, Madagas-

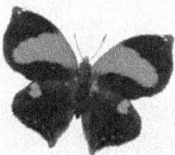

In my fiery taste and smell is a determination to make life flow more easily. I can remind you to get rid of interference in your life and to take your power back with ease and fun and without hurting anyone.

car, Zanzibar, Tanzania and the Caribbean nation Grenada.

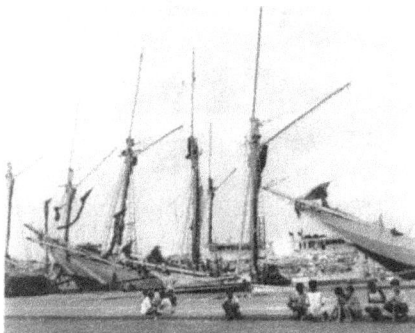

Pinisi Freighters in the port of Taopere in Makassar. Courtesy: Marc Obrowski

Parts used: Sun-dried unopened flower buds

Global summary – medicinal uses:
Used as a(n): antithelmintic (destroys intestinal parasites), carminative (enhances digestion, reduces gas and cramps), stimulant, anti-asthmatic, aphrodisiac, antiseptic, anti-fungal, anti-bacterial, anti-viral.
Used to treat: nausea, vomiting, morning sickness, male sexual dysfunction, dental pains and emergencies (clove contains eugenol, an anesthetic), oxidative stress, and hemorrhoids.

Summary medicinal uses and properties supported by scientific studies:
Essential oil of clove has been found to work as an analgesic, anti-inflammatory, antioxidant, anti-microbial, anti-fungal, anti-viral (herpes simplex –HSV I&II and hepatitis C), anti-bacterial (including a several of the multi-drug resistant Staphylococcus epidermidis), anti-cancer, cancer protective (skin and lung), anti-diabetic, and insect repellant. It contains aphrodisiac properties. A cream from clove works as an effective treatment for chronic anal fissures.

Austria - Vienna:
This study discovered more about the mechanism of how the essential oil of clove's potent anti-oxidant properties work.[1]

China - Harbin:
Scientists confirmed the anti-microbial activity of clove's essential oil against a variety of bacterial and fungal pathogens, including those of Staphylococcus epidermidis, Escherichia coli and Candida albicans.[2]

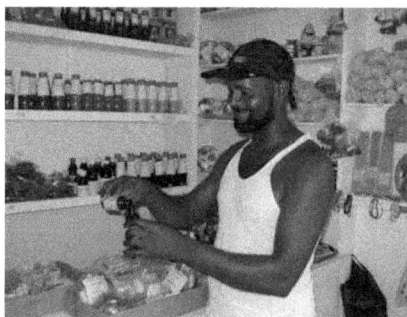

Spice vendor pouring clove oil. Grenada 2007

Egypt - Mansoura:
In an enrolled study, patients suffering from chronic anal fissures were given a clove oil 1% cream preparation. Healing occurred in five times as many patients as in the control group. The 1% clove cream patients also had a greater reduction in resting anal pressure than those in the control group.[3]

German Commission E:
Approved for oral inflammations.

India - Gujarat & Kolkata:
Aspergillus niger, a "black fungus", can become a serious health threat to humans when inhaled in large quantities and over prolonged periods of time. Essen-

tial oil of clove has been found to inhibit its growth and spore formation making it a potential treatment possibility for patients suffering from aspergillosis.[4]

One study from Kolkata looked at the properties of aqueous solution of clove and found it to produce apoptosis of lung cancer cells in mice as well as having other possible cancer protective properties.[5] Another Indian study determined that aqueous solution of clove might also have protective properties against skin papillomas (skin tumor).[6]

Clove has long had a standing reputation in the Unani traditions as an aphrodisiac for males. Now, an Aligarh Muslim University study may provide further clues as to why it works in the treatment of male sexual dysfunctions. Researchers noted that normal male rats given a 50% alcoholic extract of clove (between 100mg/kg to 500mg/kg) registered significantly enhanced sexual appetites without any noticeable side effects.

How does clove do it? Is it that by supporting the part of you that can take care of your survival needs more effectively and efficiently that energy is freed to meet your higher needs for sexual happiness?

Japan - Tokyo:

Clove preparations given orally to mice infected with oral and gastro-intestinal Candida albicans (fungus) overgrowth showed a marked reduction of fungal spread and a reduction of symptoms.[7]

In a series of experiments, Virologists from the Toyama Medical and Pharmaceutical University in Sugitani determined that eugeniine, a compound purified from the extracts of clove, inhibits viral DNA synthesis in several strains of herpes (I & II), including acyclovir-phosphonoacetic acid-resistant HSV-I.[8]

Pakistan - Karachi:

Scientists from the Department of Pharmacology at the Aga Khan University Medical College reported the result of their study: "...clove oil is inhibitory of platelet aggregation and thromboxane synthesis and may act as anti-thrombotic agent." [9]

Tunisia - Africa:

A study reported in the National Library of Medicine determined essential oil of clove extracts to have analgesic, anti-inflammatory, antioxidant, anti-microbial, anti-fungal, anti-viral (herpes simplex –HSV and hepatitis C), anti-bacterial (including several of the multi-drug resistant Staphylococcus epidermidis) and insect repellant properties.[10]

United States – Nashville:

Vanderbilt University School of Medicine scientists explored clove's ability to act as an insulin-like substance, which may prove beneficial in the treatment of diabetes.[11] The data apparently revealed that clove, much like insulin, stimulates a certain gene sequence expression and thereby sets in motion chemical reactions important in effective sugar metabolism.

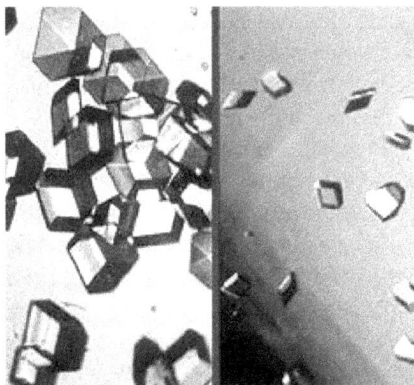

Insulin crystals. Courtesy: NASA

PREPARATIONS:

Topical: essential oil, cream, powder or diluted mouthwash.

Internal: Take ~3gm of crushed cloves pour a cup of cool water and bring to a boil. Allow to cool and drink in case of digestive difficulties such as nausea or gas.

Unwanted Effects:

Skin irritations.

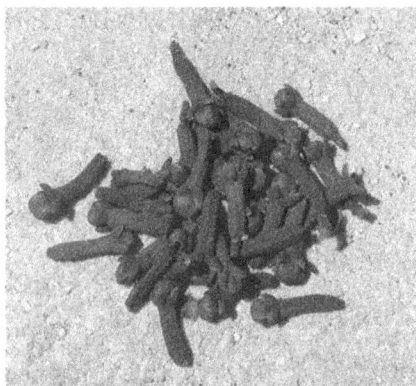

Sun dried clove buds. Grenada 2007

WARNING:

The single major active ingredient in the essential oil of clove is eugenol, which comprises almost 80% of the oil.[12] This study also determined that the oil had cytotoxic (toxic to cells) properties against fibroblasts (cells in the connective tissue producing collagen) and endothelial cells (cells that form the lining of organs) in the laboratory.

Pregnant women should avoid clove in large quantities. While clove has been used as a carminative, it has been known to irritate the gastro-intestinal tract in people with heightened sensitivity. Be especially careful if you are suffering from chronic bowel conditions such as colitis or irritable bowel syndrome (IBS).

Possible interaction with drugs:

A study from Brazil determined that the essential oil of clove, among several other plant extracts, had a significant synergistic effect along with 13 antimicrobial drugs used by doctors to treat contagious bacterial (Staphylococcus aureus strains) diseases.[13]

Clove oil reportedly possesses blood-thinning properties, suggesting wise use when taken in conjunction with other blood thinners (herbal or pharmaceutical, such as willow bark extract, ginkgo biloba or coumadin).

Also, to avoid contributing to gastrointestinal ulcer escalation, exercise caution if you take any non-steroidal anti-inflammatory (NSAID'S) drugs, especially over a longer period of time.

Overdoses of oil of clove have been reported. If you suspect a clove overdose contact your poison control center or seek immediate medical attention.

1 Jirovetz L, Buchbauer G, Stoilova I, Stoyanova A, Krastanov A, Schmidt E. *Chemical composition and antioxidant properties of clove leaf essential oil.* Department of Clinical Pharmacy and Diagnostics, University of Vienna, Althanstrasse 14, A-1090 Vienna, Austria. J Agric Food Chem. 2006 Aug 23;54(17):6303-7.

2 Fu Y, Zu Y, Chen L, Shi X, Wang Z, Sun S, Efferth T. *Antimicrobial activity of clove and rosemary essential oils alone and in combination.* Key Laboratory of Forest Plant Ecology, Ministry of Education, Northeast Forestry University, Harbin 150040, P. R. China. Phytother Res. 2007 Jun 11.

3 Elwakeel HA, Moneim HA, Farid M, Gohar AA. *Clove oil cream: a new effective treatment for chronic anal fissure.* Mansoura Faculty of Medicine, Surgery, Mansoura University Hospital, Mansoura, Dakhlia, Egypt. Colorectal Dis. 2007 Jul;9(6):549-52.

4 Pawar VC, Thaker VS. *In vitro efficacy of 75 essential oils against Aspergillus niger.* Department of Biosciences, Saurashtra Uni-

versity, Rajkot, Gujarat, India. Mycoses. 2006 Jul;49(4):316-23.

5 Banerjee S, Panda CK, Das S. *Clove (Syzygium aromaticum L.), a potential chemopreventive agent for lung cancer.* Department of Cancer Chemoprevention, Chittarajan National Cancer Institute, 37, S.P. Mukherjee Road, Kolkata 700026, India. Carcinogenesis. 2006 Aug;27(8):1645-54. Epub 2006 Feb 25.

6 Banerjee S, Das S. *Anticarcinogenic effects of an aqueous infusion of cloves on skin carcinogenesis.* Dept. of Cancer Chemoprevention, Chittarajan National Cancer Institute, 37 S.P. Mukherjee Road, Kolkata 700026, West Bengal, India. Asian Pac J Cancer Prev. 2005 Jul-Sep;6(3):304-8.

7 Taguchi Y, Ishibashi H, Takizawa T, Inoue S, Yamaguchi H, Abe S. *Protection of oral or intestinal candidiasis in mice by oral or intragastric administration of herbal food, clove (Syzygium aromaticum).* Research and Development Division, S & B Foods Inc., 38-8 Miyamoto-cho, Itabashiku, Tokyo 174-8651, Japan. Nippon Ishinkin Gakkai Zasshi. 2005;46(1):27-33.

8 Kurokawa M, Hozumi T, Basnet P, Nakano M, Kadota S, Namba T, Kawana T, Shiraki K. *Purification and characterization of eugeniin as an anti-herpesvirus compound from Geum japonicum and Syzygium aromaticum.* Virology, Toyama Medical and Pharmaceutical University, Sugitani, Toyama 930-01, Japan. J Pharmacol Exp Ther. 1998 Feb;284(2):728-35.

9 Saeed SA, Gilani AH. *Antithrombotic activity of clove oil.* Department of Pharmacology, Aga Khan University Medical College, Karachi. J Pak Med Assoc. 1994 May;44(5):112-5.

10 Chaieb K, Hajlaoui H, Zmantar T, Kahla-Nakbi AB, Rouabhia M, Mahdouani K, Bakhrouf A. *The chemical composition and biological activity of clove essential oil, Eugenia caryophyllata (Syzigium aromaticum L. Myrtaceae): a short review.* Laboratoire d'Analyses, Traitement et Valorisation des Polluants de l'Environnement et des Produits, Faculté de Pharmacie, rue Avicenne 5000 Monastir, Tunisie. Phytother Res. 2007 Jun;21(6):501-6.

11 Prasad RC, Herzog B, Boone B, Sims L, Waltner-Law M. *An extract of Syzygium aromaticum represses genes encoding hepatic gluconeogenic enzymes.* Department of Molecular Physiology and Biophysics, Vanderbilt University School of Medicine, Nashville, TN 37232, USA. J Ethnopharmacol. 2005 Jan 4;96(1-2):295-301.

12 Prashar A, Locke IC, Evans CS. *Cytotoxicity of clove (Syzygium aromaticum) oil and its major components to human skin cells.* School of Biosciences, University of Westminster, London, UK Cell Prolif. 2006 Aug;39(4):241-8.

Amharic: Krinfud
Dutch: Kruidnagel
French: Clou de girofle
German: Gewürznelke
Hebrew: Tsiporen
Hindi: Laung
Homeopathic: Syzygium jambolanum
only (Syzyg.)
Italian: Chiodo di garofano
Korean: Jeonghyang
Latin: Syzygium aromaticum
Russian: Gvozdika
Sanskrit: Lavanga
Spanish: Clavo

13 Betoni JE, Mantovani RP, Barbosa LN, Di Stasi LC, Fernandes Junior A. *Synergism between plant extract and antimicrobial drugs used on Staphylococcus aureus diseases.* Departamento de Farmacologia, Instituto de Biociências, Universidade Estadual Paulista Julio de Mesquita Filho, Botucatu, SP, 18618-000, Brasil. Mem Inst Oswaldo Cruz. 2006 Jun;101(4):387-90.

Growth: Clove is an evergreen and tropical tree, which reaches up to 40-feet high in the wild. At this size it can sprout a dense canopy about 15-feet wide.

Native to: The Indonesian Molucca islands; but is now also grown on Zanzibar, Madagascar and other parts of East Africa. The clove tree only grows within sight of the oceans. Inland propagation has failed. Clove production takes place almost entirely on islands and coastal properties.

How to grow clove: Clove trees grow from seeds or cuttings. Allow the seeds to ripen on the tree and fall on their own accord. Pick seeds, soak them over night in a container of water, and plant them the next day in a container filled with loose, rich organic soil at a depth about half an inch and about the same distance apart. Protect them from extreme sun and weather. In about two weeks the trees will begin to sprout. When the roots are well established, transplant the seedlings into larger containers and let them grow in a sheltered shady environment. Remove any unhealthy looking plants to avoid contamination. Transplant the tree about a year or two afterwards, ideally into a diverse garden that allows for partial shade. Flowers and seeds may not appear until the tree matures about five to seven years later.

Time to seed: In the summer months when the seeds begin to fall on their own accord. Do not let them lie on the ground for more than a few days. You can achieve higher germination when the seeds are freshly fallen.

Sun: Tropical sun with partial shade.

Zone: 10-11. Does well especially in costal climate in zones with temperatures between $15 - 30$ C°. It cannot handle frost conditions.

Soil: Well drained soil, with an ideally even distribution of sufficient rain.

Harvest: The buds are picked by hand just as they begin to open. Break the clusters into individual pieces, spread them in a shallow fashion onto a breathable and clean surface, and allow them to dry slowly in the sun. The complete process may take up to five days.

Attracts friends: Bees, birds, pollinating bats.

Environmental benefits: Honey collected from hives near clove trees is a specialty.

Storage: In a dry container, kept out of the sun.

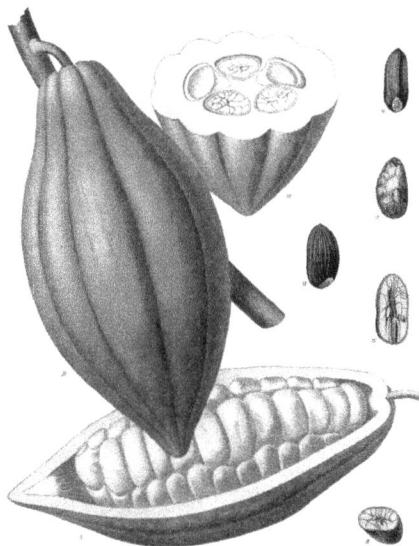

Köhler's Medicinal Plants 1887

Cocoa

To be happy is to meet your needs.

Once ancient and exotic, cocoa was called "the drink of the Gods". A reputation earned, perhaps, for the feeling produced of virility and happiness; or, because, according to one version of an Aztec legend, the Love Goddess Xochiquetzal, patron of sacred prostitutes, lovers, marriage, dancing, singing, magic and the arts, was associated with the cocoa plant; or for another version that credits Xochiquetzal's son and lover, the feathered serpent God Quetzalcóatl, with gifting it to the Aztecs. Mayan myths echo the ancient Aztec tales. It is interesting to note that Zecharia Sitchin, scholar of ancient Sumer, contends that Quetzalcóatl was none other that the Egyptian Thoth, exiled with a band of African followers[1] to the Americas about 5,000 years ago. Sculptures found in

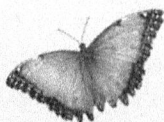

I know what I want: warm, moist weather, loose, rich soil, part sun, part shade and I do not like winds. I nurture health by balance. I am a reminder that it can be a happy pleasure to meet your needs gently and consistently. I can help to release the stress of the day and regain your natural attribute of peace.

Mexico, thought to be more than 3,000 years old, are considered by some to be remnants of that exile.

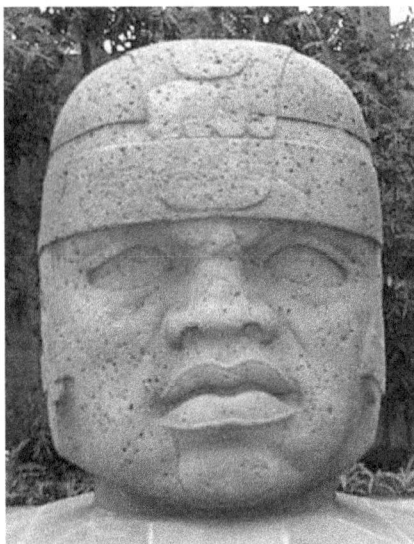

Olmec statue. Courtesy: Maunus. Museum of anthropology at Xalapa, Vera Cruz, Mexico.

Be that as it may, recent scientific studies have revealed several possible explanations for finding truths in ancient myth and common practice. Consuming cocoa releases certain chemicals such as serotonin, 'the happy molecule' into the bloodstream. Does this account for chocolate cravings often felt by women just prior to and on their menstrual cycle?

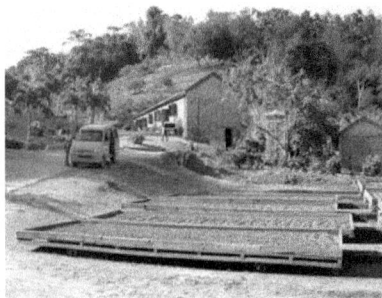

Organic cocoa plantation, Grenada. 2007

Cocoa trees are tropical plants that span the globe within a few degrees of the equator. Cocoa trees like warm, moist weather, relatively loose, rich soil and partially shaded sunlight; they dislike winds. While West Africa and Brazil have the largest cocoa plant propagation in the world, cocoa is a valuable crop in many other tropical regions, such as the spice island of Grenada.

Parts used: Bean/seed and cacao bean husk (shell)

Global summary:
Used to treat: mild asthma, high blood pressure, cough, diarrhea, diabetes, dry skin, wrinkles, pains, fatigue, low sexual virility, mild depression, and emotional discomforts.

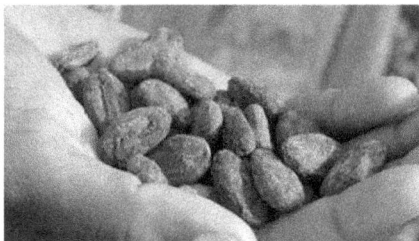

Used as a(n): Aphrodisiac, euphoric agent and mild analgesic (stimulation of certain compounds such as serotonin and dopamine), agent (tannins) to thicken gastro-intestinal content, mild stimulant (caffeine), bronchidialator (theobromine--opens of the upper parts of the lungs), muscle relaxant (smooth muscles--those in veins and intestines) and mild cardiac muscle stimulant, mild diuretic, moisturizer, and beautifier.

Cuba's traditional uses:
On the island cocoa is mostly used in traditional medicine to treat diarrhea and mild cases of asthma.

Dominican Republic

In the Dominican Republic cocoa is used as a diuretic and for kidney problems. Cacao is also used as an antiseptic, as an agent to promote menstruation, and for wound healing.

Summary medicinal uses and properties supported by scientific studies:

May balance low levels of serotonin and dopamine, enhances sexual appetite, rich in antioxidants, may play a role in the prevention of cancer, aids in atherosclerosis and heart disease, antitussive (stops cough), prevents lipid oxidation and may play a role in cholesterol homeostasis, reduces high blood pressure, photo protection, improved blood circulation, increased skin density and hydration and a decrease in skin roughness and scaling, immunomodulatory (balances immunity), inhibiting primary hemostasis (stopping the flow of blood) and pathways associated with platelet (a blood clotting component) activation and aggregation. A naturally occurring, cocoa-derived pentameric procyanidin has been shown to destroy human breast cancer cells. Cocoa bean husk extracts reduce dental plaque.

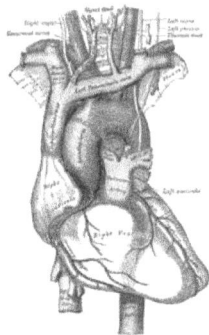

Human Heart. Grey's Anatomy 1918

Canada - Quebec:

Scientists at the McGill University School of Dietetics and Human Nutrition cautiously suggest that the consumption of dark chocolate may have protective impact on heart and vascular illness and their connection to oxidized bad cholesterol (LDL).[2]

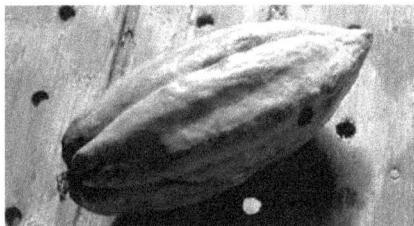

Cocoa pod. Genada 2007

England - London:

A London study looked at cocoa's component, theobromine, in the context of treating a persistent cough and determined it to be effective as an antitussive.[3]

Holland

A recent Dutch study found that the antioxidant catechin in chocolate is four times higher than that of black tea. Many in the scientific community believe that this compound may play an important part in the prevention of cancer, atherosclerosis and heart disease.

Germany - Köln:

A meta-analysis series of similar studies looking at dietary intake of cocoa and the reduction in blood pressure suggests that food rich in cocoa may contribute to a reduction of high blood pressure.[4]

Germany - Witten-Herdecke:

German scientists at the University concluded that the long-term ingestion of cocoa with a high content of flavanols provides for several markers of healthy skin: photo protection, improved blood circulation, increased skin density and hydration, and a decrease in skin roughness and scaling.[5]

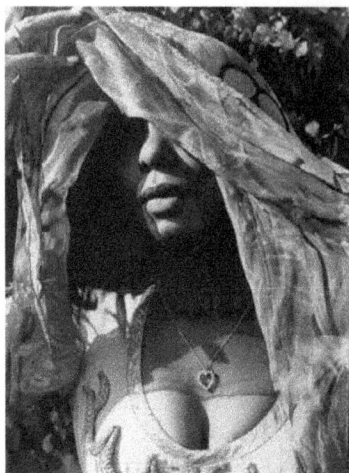
Grenadian woman, 'revealing beautiful skin'

German Commission E:

By 1991 the Commission examined the available studies on cocoa shells as therapeutic agents and determined that, at that time, there existed insufficient evidence to recommend cacao shells as a therapeutic agent.

Japan - Tokyo & Osaka

The results of this Ochanomizu University study has suggested that substances derived from cocoa powder may contribute to a reduction of bad cholesterol (LDL), an elevation of good cholesterol (HDL), and the suppression of oxidized LDL.[6]

Private Tokyo researchers found that cacao bean extract, among other compounds, has protective properties against UV-light caused wrinkle formation.[7]

Osaka University Graduate School of Dentistry researchers found that cacao bean husk extract significantly reduces plaque build up on teeth. The study confirmed the same results in vitro and in vivo.[8]

Malaysia - Selangor:

Although traditional practitioners used cocoa to work with diabetic patients, cocoa's exact working mechanism remains a mystery. However, University Putra scientists have confirmed that cocoa extract may indeed possess dose-dependent hypoglycemic and hypocholesterolemic properties.[9]

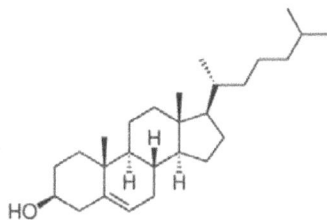
Cholesterol molecule

Switzerland - Zürich:

University Hospital doctors have summarized therapeutic properties as: antioxidant, immunomodulatory, inhibiting primary hemostasis (stopping the flow of blood) and pathways associated with platelet (a blood clotting component) activation and aggregation.[10]

United States - Chicago:

Neurologist Dr. Alan Hirsch, Director of Chicago's Smell and Taste Treatment and Research Foundation, found that people's sexual stimulation increases when exposed to the scent of chocolate.

United States - Georgetown:

Researchers at the Georgetown University Medical Center in Washington examined a cocoa-derived compound called pentameric procyanidin (pentamer) and discovered that it arrested human breast cancer cells.[11]

United States - Tuscon:

These scientists reported in a study

called 'Chocolate: Food or Drug?" that it is likely to be involved in increasing low levels of serotonin and dopamine (neurotransmitters involved in 'mood regulation.')[12]

PREPARATIONS:

Take one heaping tablespoon of organic cocoa powder and pour a cup of boiling water over it. Stir, allow it to cool and drink at the temperature to your liking.

Taking ~10gm of dark chocolate on a daily basis may lower blood pressure and reduce the risk of heart disease.

Unwanted Effects:

Cocoa is generally a very safe herb to use. In fact, it is found in most kitchens. Allergic reactions have been noted in some cases. Some times acne and headaches have been attributed to the use of chocolate. Cocoa may cause heartburn and constipation depending on dose and susceptibility. Depending on sensitivity to caffeine, it may cause the same side-effects as coffee. In some cases, children and adults with a hypersensitivity to cocoa have come down with an increased irritability, sleeplessness, restlessness and hyperactivity. Discontinue or reduce dosage if symptoms occur.

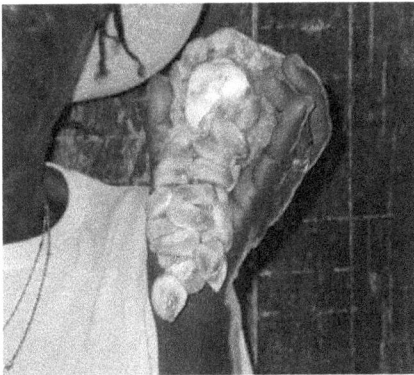

Freshly opened cocoa pod. Grenada 2007

WARNING:

A mouse study from Poland indicated that pregnant mice fed 400mg of chocolate daily produced offspring with shorter than usual limb sizes. According to their calculation a human equivalent amount of chocolate would be 200gm daily.[13] The Polish scientists advise caution when consuming large amounts of chocolate during pregnancy or when breastfeeding. It was not noted what kind of chocolate was used.

Possible interaction with drugs:

Some pharmacological drugs, such as oral contraceptives, Tagamet (blocks secretion of acid from the stomach) or even grapefruit juice, diminish the ability of the body to break down caffeine, which may cause a prolonged stimulation or 'upper' effect.

Since cocoa may contribute to reduced platelet aggregation, and thereby inhibit clotting. Be careful if you are already using blood thinners or if you have a clotting disorder.

Amharic:Amh
Dutch: Cocoa
French: Cacao
German: Kakao
Hebrew: Tsiporen
Homeopathic: Cacao (Cac.)
Italian: Cacao
Korean: Jeonghyang
Latin: Theobroma Cacao
Russian: Kakao
Spanish: Cacao

1 Sitchin, Zecharia. *The End of Days*. Harper Collins. NY. 2007.

2 Rudkowska I, Jones PJ. *Functional foods for the prevention and treatment of cardiovascular diseases: cholesterol and beyond*. School of Di-

etetics and Human Nutrition McGill University, St-Anne-de-Bellevue, Quebec, Canada. Expert Rev Cardiovasc Ther. 2007 May;5(3):477-90.

3 Usmani OS, Belvisi MG, Patel HJ, Crispino N, Birrell MA, Korbonits M, Korbonits D, Barnes PJ. *Theobromine inhibits sensory nerve activation and cough.* Department of Thoracic Medicine, National Heart and Lung Institute, Imperial College London, London, UK. FASEB J. 2005 Feb;19(2):231-3.

4 Taubert D, Roesen R, Schomig E. *Effect of cocoa and tea intake on blood pressure: a meta-analysis.* Department of Pharmacology, University Hospital of Cologne, Gleueler Strasse 24, D-50931 Cologne, Germany. Arch Intern Med. 2007 Apr 9;167(7):626-34.

5 Heinrich U, Neukam K, Tronnier H, Sies H, Stahl W. *Long-term ingestion of high flavanol cocoa provides photoprotection against UV-induced erythema and improves skin condition in women.*Institut für Experimentelle Dermatologie, Universität Witten-Herdecke, Germany. J Nutr. 2006 Jun;136(6):1565-9.

6 Baba S, Natsume M, Yasuda A, Nakamura Y, Tamura T, Osakabe N, Kanegae M, Kondo K. *Plasma LDL and HDL Cholesterol and Oxidized LDL Concentrations Are Altered in Normo- and Hypercholesterolemic Humans after Intake of Different Levels of Cocoa Powder.* Food and Health R&D Laboratories, Meiji Seika Kaisha Ltd., Saitama, 350-0289 Japan; 3Strategic Information and Ingredient Development Department, Health-care and Provisions Division, Meiji Seika Kaisha Ltd., Saitama, 104-8002 Japan 4Institute of Environmental Science for Human Life, Ochanomizu University, Tokyo, 112-8610 Japan. J Nutr. 2007 Jun;137(6):1436-1441.

7 Mitani H, Ryu A, Suzuki T, Yamashita M, Arakane K, Koide C. *Topical application of plant extracts containing xanthine derivatives can prevent UV-induced wrinkle formation in hairless mice.* Photodermatol Photoimmunol Photomed. 2007 Apr-Jun;23(2-3):86-94.

8 Matsumoto M, Tsuji M, Okuda J, Sasaki H, Nakano K, Osawa K, Shimura S, Ooshima T. *Inhibitory effects of cacao bean husk extract on plaque formation in vitro and in vivo.* Department of Pediatric Dentistry, Osaka University Graduate School of Dentistry, Osaka, Japan. Eur J Oral Sci. 2004 Jun;112(3):249-52.

9 Ruzaidi A, Amin I, Nawalyah AG, Hamid M, Faizul HA. *The effect of Malaysian cocoa extract on glucose levels and lipid profiles in diabetic rats.* Department of Nutrition and Health Sciences, Faculty of Medicine and Health Sciences, University Putra Malaysia, 43400 Serdang, Selangor, Malaysia. J Ethnopharmacol. 2005 Apr 8;98(1-2):55-60.

10 Hermann F, Ruschitzka F, Spieker L, Sudano I, Noll G, Corti R. *The sweet secret of dark chocolate.* HerzKreislaufzentrum, Kardiologie, Universitätsspital Zürich. Ther Umsch. 2005 Sep;62(9):635-7.

11 Ramljak D, Romanczyk LJ, Metheny-Barlow LJ, Thompson N, Knezevic V, Galperin M, Ramesh A, Dickson RB. *Pentameric procyanidin from Theobroma cacao selectively inhibits growth of human breast cancer cells.* Department of Oncology, The Research Building, Room W417, Lombardi Comprehensive Cancer Center, Georgetown University Medical Center, 3970 Reservoir Road, NW, Washington, District of Columbia 20057, USA. Mol Cancer Ther. 2005 Apr;4(4):537-46.

12 Bruinsma K, Taren DL. *Chocolate: food or drug?* Arizona Prevention Center, University of Arizona, College of Medicine, Tucson 85719, USA. J Am Diet Assoc. 1999 Oct;99(10):1249-56.

13 Skopiski P, Skopiska-Rózewska E, Sommer E, Chorostowska-Wynimko J, Rogala E, Cendrowska I, Chrystowska D, Filewska M, Biaas-Chromiec B, Bany J. *Chocolate feeding of pregnant mice influences length of limbs of their progeny.* Dept. Histol. Embryol. Biostructure Center, Chaubiskiego 5, 02-004 Warsaw, Poland. Pol J Vet Sci. 2003;6(3 Suppl):57-9.

Growth: Cocoa grows almost anywhere within an imaginary belt of 10° degrees North and South of the equator. The tree can reach up to 60-feet high in the wild, while most plantation trees remain near 25 feet.

How to grow cocoa: Cocoa trees prefer warmth and evenly constant, moist weather conditions common to many islands near the equator. However, they do not like windy conditions, but rather prefer sheltered ones. Cocoa provides the most potent properties of taste and therapeutics when grown in mixed organic gardens that include papaya, banana, coconuts and many other local and sustainable crops that share an affinity for similar sun, soil and weather conditions. Cocoa trees are self-pollinating.

Take a seedpod from a cocoa tree that you know has a high yield to ensure abundant future harvests. Plant them in containers filled with rich, moist, organic soil. Within a few months the baby cocoa plant will have sprouted and developed a sufficient root system that allows for a successful transplant into the ground.

Native to: Equatorial Americas; but nowadays they also grow in areas within 10° of the equator.

Time to seed: Grown from seed or from rooted branch cuttings. In the tropics where cocoa grows; the growing season is continuous.

Sun: Cocoa trees grow best as an under-story tree to larger tropical trees that allow for diffused sunlight.

Zone: In temperature zones almost anywhere within an imaginary belt of 10° degrees North and South of the equator.

Soil: Loose, moist, rich soil.

Harvest: The tropical cocoa tree carries fruit throughout the year and is harvested twice a year. Only the ripe fruit is picked - which takes some experience.

Attracts friends: Bees.

Environmental benefits and concerns: Since cocoa trees do best as an under-story tree, the tree promotes the existence of large canopy trees that together provide a natural biodiversity and environment for other plant and animal.

The plant itself also seems stronger in organic mixed environments that allow for natural and self-balancing pest control. Larger plantations are often hounded by pest problems that can destroy large portions of plantation in a relatively short amount of time.

Storage: The ripe pods are harvested, cut open and the seeds are extracted and poured into bins which are covered completely with fresh banana leaves. The seeds are left there for a few days (2-5) to ferment, which produces a significant amount of heat that you can easily feel by touching the leaves. The fermentation brings about the cocoa flavor. After this process completes, place single layers of the seeds on trays, exposing them to the sun until completely dried. Quickly cover the trays in the event of sudden tropical rain. Finally, sort by size and de-shell, roast and ground into a thick liquid. Extract the cocoa butter and cocoa powder - the raw materials for chocolate and a host of other products.

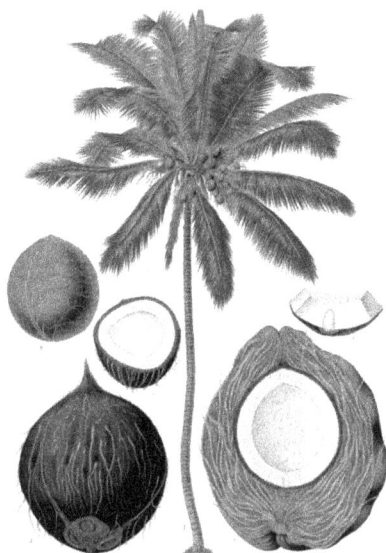

Köhler's Medicinal Plants 1887

Coconut

Just Enjoy

The windswept swaying and elegance of coconut trees adds an exotic tropical beauty to almost any painting of a South Sea island or a Micronesia atoll. Coconut is truly an old friend of humanity and an indispensable character in adventure movies and pirate novels alike. Its exact origin is not clearly known. While not considered a spice at all, I wanted to include it here because coconut offers more than a wonderful beverage companion to spicy foods. Coconut fits perfectly with the principle of this book when examining natural, effective, safe and affordable medicines. This useful tree's numerous parts serve millions of people around the world and are employed in any form of traditional medicine where the plant is present. On one hand, coconut acts as an impor-

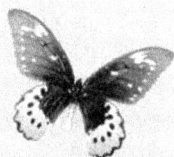

I offer shelter from the storm. I bring energy to those that are tired. I provide sweet sustenance to feed your body. I give soothing relief for much what ails you. I am a living reminder that you too can live in a world where trust is the breath that gives rise to your happiness. That breath offers a life to having your needs be met as easy as my leaves sway in the warm ocean breeze.

tant partner in producing health, healing and a desired level of energy. On the other hand, it provides help in meeting our needs for beauty, shelter, and nutritional food. In much of Northern India, coconut is used extensively in Ayurvedic medicine. In Tamil Nadu, the tradition of Siddha uses coconut, as do many of the Arabian countries within their Unani tradition. It almost goes without saying that the Maori from New Zealand and other islanders reaching from Hawaii to the South Seas and across to Micronesia use coconut for medicinal purposes. Here in the city of Accra, Ghana fresh coconut is served as an energizing, liquid lunch and refreshment on almost every street corner for nothing but a quarter.

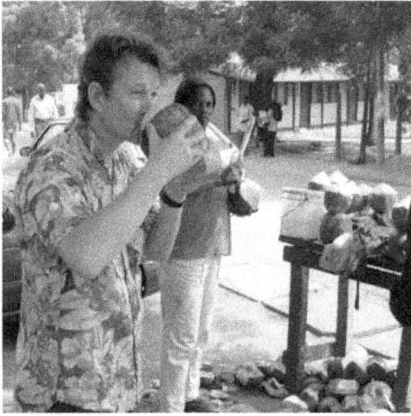

Coconut vendor in Accra, Ghana 2008
Photo by Jojo Quayson

Parts used: Coconut water (a clear liquid of younger, unripe nuts), fat, oil, meat (the inner white layer of the seed), coconut milk (pulp boiled in sweet, milky water), khopra (dried and grated coconut meat), palm sugar, sap and coconut flower as a gluten free alternative to wheat.

Global summary:
Used to treat: Used to treat: arthritis, asthma, allergies, bronchitis, cough, colds and flu, pharyngitis (sore throat), thyroid problems, tuberculosis, constipation, diarrhea, inflammatory bowel disease (IBD), liver and gall bladder problems, gastro-intestinal ulcers, nausea and vomiting, hemorrhoids, certain parasites, diabetes, obesity, food (carbohydrate) craving, insomnia, irritability, ear infections, fever, fungal infections, certain venereal diseases, vaginal dryness, vaginal yeast infection, lice and scabies, cancer and tumors, malnutrition, low immunity, skin problems (psoriasis, ulcers, abscess, poorly healing wounds, rash, burns, rosacea, dryness, itching), inflammation, wrinkles, age-spots, sunburn, fatigue, low libido and generalized weakness. May prevent: heart disease, atherosclerosis, high blood pressure and stroke.
Used as a(n): anti-bacterial, anti-fungal, anti-parasitical, anti-viral, 'pick me up', source of multiple nutrients, immune supporter, skin protector, moisturizer and lubricant, antioxidant, anti-inflammatory and multiple system tonics.

Summary medicinal uses and properties supported by scientific studies:
Anti-bacterial (e.g. gonorrhea, staphylococcus aureus, chlamydia), anti-fungal (Candida albicans), anti-viral (e.g. herpes, visna virus), an aide in cholesterol homeostasis, possible weight loss agent, possible protective against ischemic heart disease, protects liver from alcohol-induced damage and may also protect against endotoxemia (the presence of toxic material from the inside of bacteria in the blood that can lead to organ failure, shock and even death).

Iceland - Reykjavík:

'In this study from Iceland researchers discovered in a laboratory experiment that medium chain fatty acids, but especially capric acid ($C_{10}H_{20}O_2$), worked effectively in killing all strains of Neisseria gonorrhea.'[1]

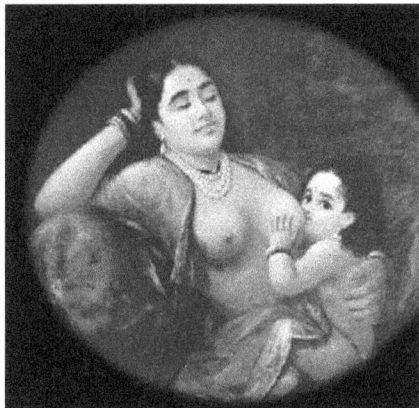

Raja Ravi Varma (1848-1906) India

Did you know that lauric acid ($C_{12}H_{24}O_2$), which is the main medium chain fatty acid in coconut oil, is also found in high concentrations in mother's milk? It has known anti-viral properties that are capable of dismantling the viral envelope thereby causing its demise. Among the tested viruses was the common herpes virus. Capric acid is contained in smaller amounts of coconut oil and is a close relative to lauric acid. Chemical similarities between coconut milk and mother's milk echo a shared therapeutic value.

Iceland - Reykjavík:

Another laboratory study from the island determined how well medium chain fatty acids destroy or inhibit the growth of other groups of bacteria. Both lauric acid and capric acid showed strong anti-bacterial abilities.[2]

Iceland - Reykjavík:

Again researchers demonstrated another aspect of lauric and capric acids broad anti-microbial properties in the laboratory; this time against a fungus associated with yeast infections.[3]

Iceland - Reykjavík:

Lauric acid and capric acid were also found to effectively inactivate Chlamydia in the laboratory. This suggests, that these two fatty acids, found in relatively high concentrations in coconut milk and fat, may play a role in the prevention of this particular bacterial infection as well.[4]

United States - Staten Island:

The authors of this study state: "Lipids can inactivate enveloped viruses, bacteria, fungi, and protozoa." By adding medium chain fatty acids (MCFA) to HIV-infected blood products the researchers learned that they could reduce the virus concentration by a very large number. Furthermore, the scientists expect that MCFA "…may potentially be used as combination spermicidal and virucidal agents."[5]

Sri Lanka - Ragama:

The people of the island nation Sri Lanka, like many other tropical islanders, use coconut oil as a main source for their oil and fat needs. Different than other saturated fats, the medium chain fatty acids in unprocessed virgin coconut oil are easily digested and quickly converted into energy.[6]

India - Kerala:

This interesting study found that cholesterol-fed rats that were given coconut water from either tender or mature coconuts significantly reduced general cholesterol and bad cholesterol (LDL), but increased good cholesterol (HDL).[7]

India – Kerala:
The authors of another combination laboratory-animal study from the same university wrote that: "…The results demonstrated the potential beneficiary effect of virgin coconut oil in lowering lipid levels in serum and tissues and LDL oxidation by physiological oxidants."[8]

Japan – Yamanashi:
Based on the well-established observation that MCFA (present in coconut) are able to prevent alcohol induced liver damage, these researchers established that eating MFCA might also protect the liver from endotoxins[9] (toxic material inside of bacteria which are released when the bacteria is destroyed, sometimes called 'die-off' reaction).

North Carolina – USA:
Mary L. Moore, an associate Professor in the Department of Obstetrics and Gynecology at the Wake Forest University School of Medicine in Winston-Salem, discovered in recent meta-analysis research on the benefits of breast feeding that babies who are breast fed have a reduced level of total and LDH cholesterol in their later adult life.[10]

Canada – Quebec:
These nutritional scientists examined the ability of medium chain fatty acids to convert quickly into energy. They concluded, based on their laboratory examinations and meta-analysis in animal and human trials, that MCFA 'may be used as a means to produce weight loss.'[11]

United States – New York:
Researcher Hans Kaunitz correlates the data from several laboratory animal studies with the findings from the United Nations and reports on some possible reasons that death from ischemic heart disease is lowest where the coconut fat intake is the highest.[12]

PREPARATIONS:
United States – Princeton:
This meta-analysis led these researchers to note that: "The safety of human dietary consumption of medium chain triglycerides up to levels of 1g/kg has been confirmed in several clinical trials."[13]

Cuban Santeros use coconut frequently as part of complex initiation ceremonies.

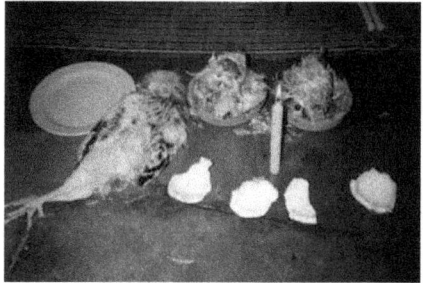

Coconut flesh are part of the offerings to the ancient Orishas. Havana, Cuba

For general health and prevention take a tablespoon of organic coconut oil with food or a beverage twice a day.

For more chronic conditions consider 2 tablespoons twice daily with food or a beverage.

Coconut water; direct from the nut - drink as much as you like.

I case of head lice, cover the scalp with coconut oil, wear a shower cap over night wash and rinse in the morning.

To reduce the feeling of hunger, take one teaspoon of organic, virgin coconut oil about a half an hour before a meal.

To ease constipation and hemorrhoidal conditions take a teaspoon before retiring at night.

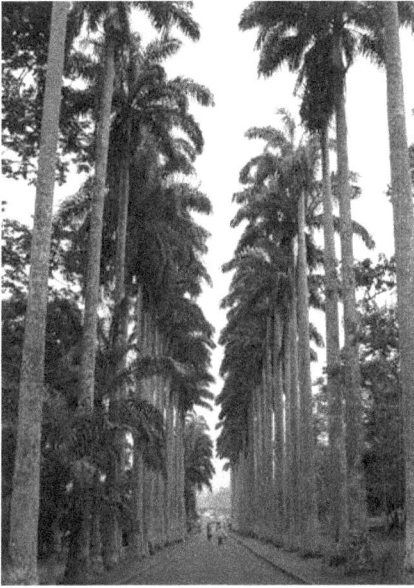

Coconut trees. Aburi Botanical Gardens, Ghana. 2008

CONSIDER:

If you fear an increase in cholesterol but want to try working with coconut oil, consider a frequent cholesterol panel to monitor your progress.

Possible interaction with drugs:

None known.

1 Bergsson G, Steingrímsson O, Thormar H. *In vitro susceptibilities of Neisseria gonorrhoeae to fatty acids and monoglycerides*. Institute of Biology, University of Iceland. gudmunb@ rhi.hi.is Antimicrob Agents Chemother. 1999 Nov;43(11):2790-2.

2 Bergsson G, Arnfinnsson J, Steingrímsson O, Thormar H. *Killing of Gram-positive cocci by fatty acids and monoglycerides*. Institute of Biology, University of Iceland, Reykjavik. gudmunb@hi.is APMIS. 2001 Oct;109(10):670-8.

3 Bergsson G, Arnfinnsson J, Steingrímsson O ,

Thormar H. *In vitro killing of Candida albicans by fatty acids and monoglycerides*. Institute of Biology, University of Iceland, Reykjavik, Iceland. gudmunb@hi.is Antimicrob Agents Chemother. 2001 Nov; 45(11):3209-12.

4 Bergsson G, Arnfinnsson J, Karlsson SM, Steingrímsson O, Thormar H. In vitro inactivation of Chlamydia trachomatis by fatty acids and monoglycerides. Institute of Biology, University of Iceland, Reykjavik, Iceland. Antimicrob Agents Chemother. 1998 Sep;42(9):2290-4.

5 Isaacs CE, Kim KS, Thormar H. Inactivation of enveloped viruses in human bodily fluids by purified lipids. Department of Developmental Biochemistry, New York State Institute for Basic Research in Developmental Disabilities, Staten Island 10314. Ann N Y Acad Sci. 1994 Jun 6;724:457-64.

6 Amarasiri WA, Dissanayake AS. Coconut fats. Department of Physiology, Faculty of Medicine, University of Kelaniya, Ragama, Sri Lanka. Ceylon Med J. 2006 Jun;51(2):47-51.

7 V.G. Sandhya, Dr., Professor T. Rajamohan. Beneficial Effects of Coconut Water Feeding on Lipid Metabolism in Cholesterol-Fed Rats. Journal of Medicinal Food. Sep 2006, Vol. 9, No. 3: 400-407

8 Nevin KG, Rajamohan T. Beneficial effects of virgin coconut oil on lipid parameters and in vitro LDL oxidation. Department of Biochemistry, University of Kerala, Kariavattom, Thiruvananthapuram 695 581, India. Clin Biochem. 2004 Sep;37(9):830-5.

9 Kono H, Fujii H, Asakawa M, Yamamoto M, Matsuda M, Maki A, Matsumoto Y. Protective effects of medium-chain triglycerides on the liver and gut in rats administered endotoxin. First Department of Surgery, Yamanashi Medical University, Yamanashi, Japan. hkouno@res.yamanashi-med.ac.jp Ann Surg. 2003 Feb;237(2):246-55.

10 Moore ML. Current studies on two separate topics: breastfeeding postpartum length of hospital stay. Department of Obstetrics and Gynecology at the Wake Forest University School of Medicine in Winston-Salem, North Carolina. J Perinat Educ. 2003 Spring;12(2):44-6.

11 Papamandjaris AA, MacDougall DE, Jones PJ. Medium chain fatty acid metabolism and energy expenditure: obesity treatment implica-

tions. School of Dietetics and Human Nutrition, Faculty of Agricultural and Environmental Sciences, McGill University, Macdonald Campus, Ste-Anne-de-Bellevue, Quebec. Life Sci. 1998;62(14):1203-15.

12 Kaunitz H. Medium chain triglycerides (MCT) in aging and arteriosclerosis.J Environ Pathol Toxicol Oncol. 1986 Mar-Apr;6(3-4):115-21.

13 Traul KA, Driedger A, Ingle DL, Nakhasi D. Review of the toxicologic properties of medium-chain triglycerides. Ingle & Traul Pharmaceutical Consulting, Inc., PO Box 2152, Princeton, NJ 08543, USA. katraul@aol.com Food Chem Toxicol. 2000 Jan;38(1):79-98.

Amharic: Kokonet
Dutch: Kokosnoot
French: Noix de coco
German: Kokosnuß
Hawaiian: Niu
Hebrew: Kokus
Hindi: Narial
Homeopathic: Cocos nucifera
              (Coco-n.)
Italian: Cocco
Korean: Kokosu
Latin: Cocos nucifera L.
Russian: Kokos
Sanskrit: Naarikela
Spanish: Coco fruto
Swahili: Nazi

Growth: The coconut is a tropical tree can reach to up to 100 feet.

Native to: Scientists contest the exact origin of the coconut tree.

How to grow coconut: Choose a ripe and fallen, brown and wrinkly looking coconut with its outer shell intact. Soak it in a container of water for three days. Use a 3-5 gallon pot. Fill the pot with a few rocks at the bottom for good drainage, and top it off with 2/3 rich organic soil mixed with 1/3 sand. Place the coconut halfway deep into the pot - pretty much the way you found it on the ground. Now the nut is covered half by soil, while the other half is exposed to the air. Find a warm spot with sun and partial shade. Begin watering the nut daily with lukewarm water keeping it constantly moist but not wet to produce germination. This requires patience and diligence. Think of it as your baby that needs daily care. Too much water will rot the nut, while not enough water results in stagnation. The whole process may take several months for signs of life to appear. Some coconuts begin sprouting on top, while others begin shooting roots. Once the plant has solidly taken, you can transplant it to its permanent spot. You can use organic fertilizer from compost to nurture the tree into maturity.

Time to seed: The coconut is a tough nut. It is able to survive long voyages on the salty ocean seas and sprout when washed ashore thousands of miles away. In a native climate anytime.

Sun: Initially partial shade and later full sun to partial shade.

Zone: 10 – 11.

Soil: The coconut can thrive in a great variety of soil types as long as sufficient water, proper microorganisms and nutrients are available.

Harvest: As soon as the nut appears, matures and falls by itself, which may take several years.

Attracts friends: Coconut crabs are not just the largest hermit crabs in the world but they are also the only animal that is able to cut open a coconut and consume its content.

Environmental benefits: Virtually every part of the tree is used in a myriad of natural products produced by mom and pop family businesses as well by larger industries; from food to medicines, from household articles, building materials to charcoal. The list of coconut-related products is perhaps longer than that of any other tree.

Storage: Coconuts can be stored for long periods, conserving coconut water and flesh.

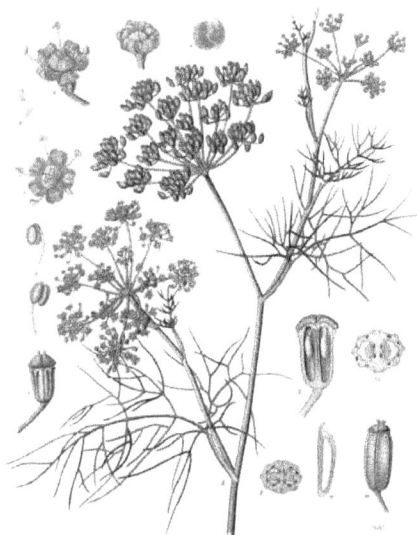

Köhler's Medicinal Plants 1887

Fennel

I am light, my stem is filled with space yet I am naturally strong and beautiful.

Fennel, an aerie aromatic plant, can reach up to 2.5 m (7-8ft.) in height. For more than 3,000 years, fennel has provided a home to various butterfly species as well as offering fruits (seeds) and leaves for food, aroma and medicine. While most ancient records related to fennel derive from the Mediterranean region and North Africa, the plant can be found today along most of the same latitude having established itself further north and south. It is now common in northern America, northern Europe, southern Canada and has actually become a weed problem in Australia.

Fennel is often mistaken for cumin, caraway, anise and even licorice. While the scent may be similar caraway and anise have white flowers, cumin blooms pink and fennel yellow, licorice looks al-

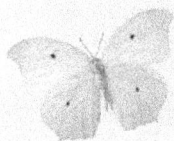

My scent is sweet and refreshing and I love myself. I hope to remind you that strength and power comes in many shapes. I am happy with what I am and when you touch my scent and swallow my fruit perhaps you can accept and love your unique shape, powers and abilities, your unique bodies and their special movements and patterns of creations. Eat me and let all this be a part of you.

together different, and, instead of using the fruits as with the other three, its root is primarily used. The dried fennel fruit, generally light green, retains its color especially when grown organically.

Parts used: Ripe fruit, dried fruit, fresh leaves and oil.

Global summary:
Used to treat: bad breath, eye infection, dysmenorrhea, nervousness, abdominal distention, mild abdominal cramps due to flatulence as well as to reduce phlegm in the upper respiratory tracts, especially in children. It is also used as a tea or gargle to prevent and treat bad breath.

Used as a(n): antispasmodic, carminative, antiseptic, antitussive (relieving cough), tonic, calming agent, pain reducing agent during menstrual complaints, breast enhancement, and to facilitate milk production.

Cuba's traditional uses:
Santeros (Santeria priests) use the strong-smelling fennel to counteract an ill-willed spell. It is a common ingredient in funeral ceremonies.

Germany - Hildegard von Bingen:
The famous abbess used fennel fruits and similar oils as recommended by the German Commission E. Treatments with fennel included cases of dyspepsia and catarrh of the upper respiratory tract, eye infections, low energy, and bad breath. She writes in her manuscript that to eat fennel fresh or dried makes for happiness, brings warmth and a healthy sweat, and produces an effective digestion.

Summary medicinal uses and properties supported by scientific studies:

Anti-oxidant, anti-ulcer (stomach), dysmenorrhea (menstrual pain and difficulties), colic (in infants) and hirsutism (females growing hair like a male).

Cuba's clinical uses:
Promotes appetite, relieves discomfort from gas and flatulence.

German Commission E:
Fennel seeds and oil are approved for the treatment of: "Dyspepsia such as mild, spastic gastrointestinal afflictions, fullness, flatulence. Catarrh of the upper respiratory tract."

India - Karnataka:
This study looked at the pharmacological basis for employing fennel extract in the treatment of cognitive dysfunction associated with dementia and Alzheimer's. A mouse model's results indicated that fennel extract: "...ameliorated the amnesic effect of scopolamine (0.4 mg/kg) and aging-induced memory deficits in mice."[1] These results perhaps warrant more studies using fennel extract as a therapeutic agent for such conditions.

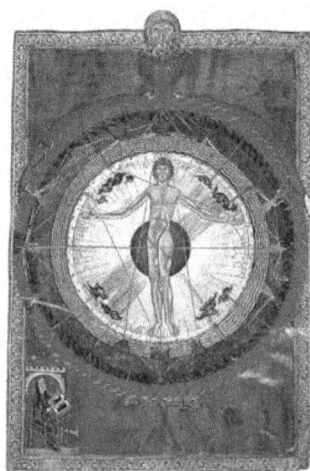

Hildegard von Bingen Manuscript ca. 1165

Iran - Kerman:

Fennel extract was found to be a more potent pain relief agent than mefenamic acid (such as Ponstel) in primary dysmenorrheal of high-school girls whose age averaged 13. In fact, it proved so effective that 80% of the fennel group no longer needed to rest in order to cope with the aches and pains.[2] Fennel is a safe plant to use, while mefenamic acid can produce serious side effects.

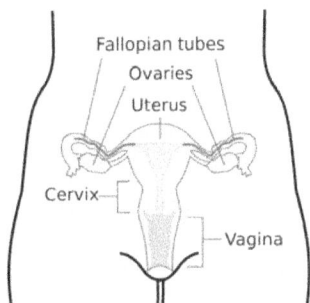

Female reproductive organs. Courtesy: CDC

Iran - Shiraz:

Fennel has been used as an estrogenic agent by traditional healers for centuries. Now scientists are looking at fennel's ability to help women who have developed hirsutism (growing hair like a male) even though they have normal menstrual cycles and normal levels of sex hormones. Researchers noted significant male type hair growth reduction when compared to the placebo. Of the two tested formulas (1% and 2%) 2% topical fennel extract proved most effective.[3]

Italy - Torino:

This study concluded that fennel extract aided with breast fed infants who had developed colic. When compared to the placebo group, those infants who had received the plant extract had a significant reduction in crying time. No side effects were noted.[4]

The phyto-estrogen like properties of fennel make it an important plant for women's health but can it also be helpful for males?

Turkey - Afyon:

These veterinary scientists confirmed some of fennel's time proven applications. Researchers confirmed its beneficial use as a treatment for digestive problems by exploring fennel's ulcer protective properties, which might be due in part to anti-oxidant properties that reduce lipid peroxidation.[5]

Another study from Turkey concluded that the essential oil of fennel protected rats from chemically induced liver damage,[6] lending credibility to fennel's reputation as a useful agent for gastro-intestinal disorders.

PREPARATIONS:

Cuban Preparation: Eight to twelve grams of crushed or ground fruit (seeds) to one liter of boiling water, and simmer for fifteen to twenty minutes. One cup (8 ounces) three times a day promotes appetite and relieves discomfort from gas and flatulence.

German Preparation: To prepare a tea, take one teaspoon of crushed dried fruits per cup of hot water, let it simmer for about 5 minutes and drink several cups a day.

Unwanted Effects:

A study from Switzerland examined three patients who had developed seizure activities apparently after using essential oils. Among the oils considered as a possible culprit for the seizures was essential oil of fennel.[7] It is thought that perhaps the intense monoterpene ketones contained in the essential oils of several different kinds of plants might be able to induce a neurological event such as a seizure.

WARNING:
Limit intake to no more than three days and do not drink during pregnancy. Do not use if allergic to fennel.

Possible interaction with drugs:
As always, be especially careful when using the concentrated essential oils. Avoid the oils on infants and when pregnant. Test for sensitivity by applying a bit to the skin of your forearm. If a reaction occurs, do not use at all. Since fennel has estrogen-like qualities, it may enhance the effects of drugs containing estrogen and hormone sensitive states such as pregnancies.

Amharic: Kamun
Italian: Finocchio
Dutch: Venkel
Korean: Pennel
French: Fenouil
Latin: Foeniculum vulgare
German: Fenchel
Russian: Fenkhel
Hebrew: Shusmar
Sanskrit: Madhurika
Hindi: Moti saunf
Spanish: Hinojo
Homeopathic: Foeniculum vulgare
        (Foen-v.)
Swahili: Shamari

1 Joshi H, Parle M. Cholinergic basis of memory-strengthen*ing effect of Foeniculum vulgare Linn.* Department of Pharmacognosy, SET's College of Pharmacy, Dharwad, Karnataka, India. J Med Food. 2006 Fall;9(3):413-7.

2 Modaress Nejad V, Asadipour M. *Comparison of the effectiveness of fennel and mefenamic acid on pain intensity in dysmenorrhoea.* Department of Obstetrics and Gynaecology, Kerman University of Medial Sciences and Health Services, Kerman, Islamic Republic of Iran. East Mediterr Health J. 2006 May-Jul;12(3-4):423-7.

3 Javidnia K, Dastgheib L, Mohammadi Samani S, Nasiri A. *Antihirsutism activity of Fennel (fruits of Foeniculum vulgare) extract.* A double-blind placebo controlled study. Faculty of Pharmacy, Shiraz University of Medical Sciences, Shiraz, Iran. javidniak@sums.ac.ir Phytomedicine. 2003;10(6-7):455-8.

4 Savino F, Cresi F, Castagno E, Silvestro L, Oggero R. *A randomized double-blind placebo-controlled trial of a standardized extract of Matricariae recutita, Foeniculum vulgare and Melissa officinalis (ColiMil) in the treatment of breastfed colicky infants.* Dipartimento di Scienze Pediatriche e dell'Adolescenza-Università di Torino, Ospedale Infantile Regina Margherita, Azienda Ospedaliera OIRM S. ANNA, Piazza Polonia, 94, 10126 Torino, Italy. Phytother Res. 2005 Apr;19(4):335-40.

5 Birdane FM, Cemek M, Birdane YO, Gülçin I, Büyükokurolu ME. *Beneficial effects of Foeniculum vulgare on ethanol-induced acute gastric mucosal injury in rats.* Department of Pharmacology, Faculty of Veterinary Medicine, Afyon Kocatepe University, Afyon, Turkey. World J Gastroenterol. 2007 Jan 28;13(4):607-11.

6 Ozbek H, Ura S, Dülger H, Bayram I, Tuncer I, Oztürk G, Oztürk A. *Hepatoprotective effect of Foeniculum vulgare essential oil.* Yüzüncü Yil University, Faculty of Medicine, Department of Pharmacology, Van 65300, Turkey. Fitoterapia. 2003 Apr;74(3):317-9.

7 Burkhard PR, Burkhardt K, Haenggeli CA, Landis T. *Plant-induced seizures: reappearance of an old problem.* Department of Neurology, University Hospital, CH-1211 Geneva 14, Switzerland, Pierre.Burkhard@hcuge.ch J Neurol. 1999 Aug;246(8):667-70.

Growth: Fennel is a perennial plant that can grow up to 4-7 feet in height.

Native to: Mediterranean but found worldwide where climate is somewhat similar.

How to grow fennel: Save some seeds from your last harvest and, after the last frost, sow them directly into your garden where you have full sun and well-drained soil. Cover the seeds lightly with a thin layer of soil approximately 1/8 to 1/4 inch deep and about a foot apart. Keep the soil only slightly moist until the first sign of growth appears. Fennel is easy to grow once geminated and needs very little attention or watering.

Time to seed: Late spring, after frost has passed. The plant is self-seeding once established.

Sun: Full Sun but can tolerate some shade.

Zone: 5 – 10

Soil: Regular soil, well drained, may add some organic compost

Harvest: Root bulbs, leafs and seeds (fresh and dried). Harvest seeds when they turn brown and dry. Rub them off the flower-stems and collect in a brown paper bag and store them in a dark and dry place. The leaves can be picked anytime once the plant is big enough to sustain a partial picking. Dig up the root, clear off the soil wash and use fresh or dry.

Attracts friends: Spittlebugs, butterflies, hummingbirds, bees, ladybugs, lacewing, hoverflies, parasitic mini wasps and big-eyed bugs.

Environmental benefits: Fast growing plant for fragrance and flowers, shelter for beneficial garden insects, natural pest control and soil erosion prevention. Fennel fragrance has been reported to repel fleas.

Food: The leaves can be used in salads, to flavor sandwiches and soups. The stems can be cut like coins and be added to salads and soups or eaten raw. Bulbs are used in many stews and soups. Seeds can be added to spreads, cheeses and breads.

Storage: Fennel bulb and leaf is best used fresh but can keep for a few days covered in a plastic bag placed in the refridgerator. Dried seeds are kept in glass with a tight lid. Color and properties remain stronger if kept out of the light.

Caution: Do not mistake fennel with poison hemlock (Conium maculatum), which while there are similarities between the plants hemlock has purple spots or streaks especially at the bottom of the stems also called the 'blood of Socrates' after the legend that tells of hemlock being used to poison the ancient philosopher. The leaves of hemlock are flat while those of fennel are fine like a needle. Hemlock also has a distinct 'musty' smell to it while fennel smells much like anise. So, if in doubt trust your nose and your eyes. Toxic doses of hemlock function as a muscle paralyser. Once the diaphragm and heart muscle are affected death can occur.

Worlds of Healing

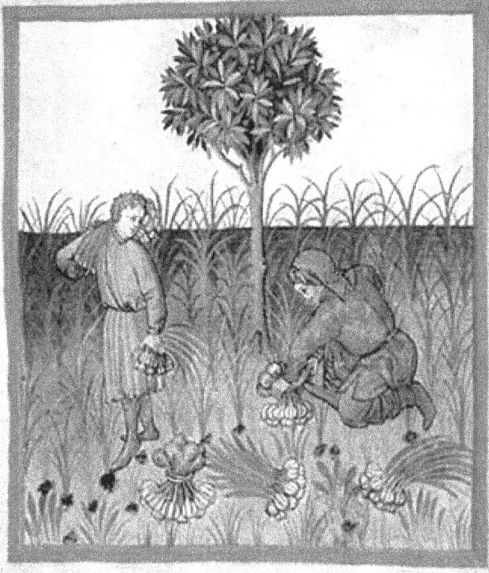

Harvesting garlic, Tacuinum sanitatis, 15th century.
Paris, Biblioteque Nationale.

Garlic

Life supports
you and loves
you totally.

Garlic, a member of the onion family, has never claimed a true place of origin. We do know, however, that many cultures have made use of this pungent bulb for thousands of years. Historical records indicate that it was used in ancient Egypt as both food and medicine. In the Histories of Herodotus, the author, considered the father of historical writing and an eyewitness from B.C., explains how machines lifted the stones of the pyramid and workers operating the machines regularly ate garlic, onions and radishes as part of their diet.[1]

For ages, many have considered garlic a virtual pharmacy. This broad international knowledge-base has not gone unnoticed by modern scientists trying to unlock the how's and why's of garlic's therapeutic properties. The

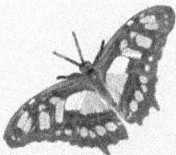

My strong flavor, my intense and lingering scent can stimulate the memory that it is okay to embrace all of you including those parts that upon first glance stink and often at a deeper look tend to have an important purpose. You too can be resilient and strong. When you taste me, when you let me, it won't be long until your blood and your joy flow more easily and freely through your veins and through your emotions. I can then assist you in releasing joy-destroying judgments and in expelling life-sucking parasites.

National Library of Health has almost 2,000 studies listed reporting on trials trying to discover its 'secrets.'

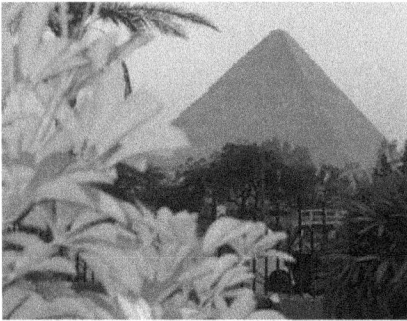

The Great Pyramid. Cairo, Egypt 2006

Parts used: Cloves

Global summary:
Used to treat: Viral, bacterial, fungal and parasitical infections (malaria prevention and treatment). Back pains, strains, inflammation, pain, sinus and bronchial congestion, asthma, fluid retention, arteriosclerosis, varicose veins and clots of all kinds, high blood pressure, arthritis, bronchitis, high cholesterol, ear infections and fever. Non-urgent allergies. Fresh garlic juice has been found to arrest the vaginal discharge from yeast infections. It is applied topically to treat burns. It is also used as a tonic and to rejuvenate sexual appetite.

Used as a(n): Tonic, expectorant, anti-asthmatic, protector of small vessels, anti-pilemic, anti-thrombolitic (prevents clods - blood thinner), anti-spasmodic, diuretic, anti-fungal, analgesic, anti-hemorrhoidal, anti-viral, anti-bacterial, anti-amoebic, anti-parasitic, anti-hypertensive.

Cuba's traditional uses:
Lumbago (rheumatic pain of the lower back), syphilis, tuberculosis, and other lung infections, as well as the loss of appetite.

Summary medicinal uses and properties supported by scientific studies from 2006-2007:
Possesses cardiovascular protective agents. May reduce risk of heart attacks in diabetic patients by contributing to better metabolic control involving blood sugar and triglycerides. Acts as an anti-oxidant, possible radioprotection (protects against damage from ionizing radiation). Able to reduce blood glucose level and reduce memory loss in Alzheimer's. Garlic is anti-microbial, anti-viral, anti-bacterial, anti-parasitical (including malaria) and anti-fungal. In addition, garlic has shown that it can produce the destruction of various cancer cells in vitro and vivo.

Cuba's clinical uses:
Garlic is one of Cuba's most versatile herbs, used for the treatment of asthma to bring up phlegm, to prevent and treat infections caused by bacteria, and decrease water retention, spasms and thrombophlebitis. Used to treat fungal infections, garlic also works as a tonic, promotes healthy veins, and prevents parasites, inflammation, hemorrhoids, bacterial infections, viral infections, hypertension, muscular pains, back pains, synovitis (inflammation of a membrane in the knee joint) and varicose veins.

German Commission E:
Approved as a treatment for: "Supportive to dietary measures at elevated levels of lipids in blood. Preventative measures for age-dependent vascular changes."

Hong Kong:
Using a rodent model, scientists reported

for the first time the high level of success obtained in inhibiting primary tumor formation of the prostrate and a reduction of secondary tumor formation. In this study garlic has shown to have potent anti-metastasis (spreading of cancer to other than the primary site) properties, which these scientists believe may also apply to other types of cancer.[2]

India - New Delhi:
In this 1996 study, scientists discovered that orally administered garlic extract for 5 consecutive days at dosages of 125, 250 and 500 mg kg-1 body weight reduced the damage to the rodents' chromosomes from gamma rays, a potent mutagenic or cancer producing agent.[3]

Italy - Ferrara:
Allicin (allylthiosulfinate, diallyl disulfide-S-monoxide), a potent, well known and researched anti-microbial and anti-fungal is an active ingredient in garlic. This laboratory study determined that concentrations of spray-dried garlic (1.5 g per 10 mL) had the strongest fungicidal reaction of those tested.[4]

Japan - Tokyo & Sakuyo:
For the first time, Japanese scientists have been able to scientifically prove what many traditional practitioners have suspected, that garlic, or specifically allicin, has potent antioxidant properties.[5]

Another study from Japan suggests that odorless garlic powder can play a beneficial role in preventing destructive thrombus (clod) formation such as in heart attacks. It apparently does so, according to the researchers, by suppressing the formation of clots and by destroying fibrin, a protein involved in the clotting of blood.[6]

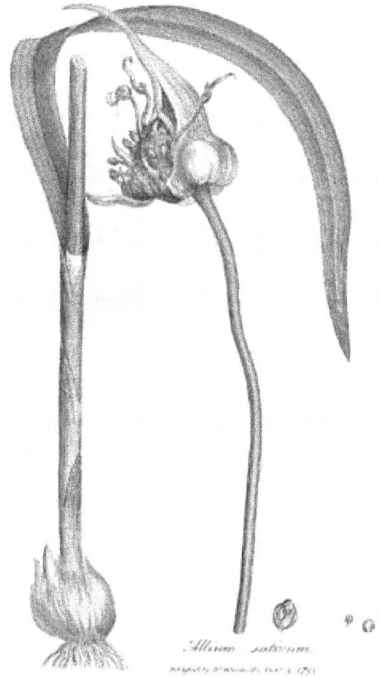

William Woodville: "Medical botany", London, James Phillips, 1793, Vol. 3

Poland - Gdask:
This study summarizes how certain compounds contained in garlic prevent and protect against cancer in vivo and in vitro. The anticancer effect of garlic is attributed to its organosulfuric compounds.[7] Furthermore, this study noted that population based case studies indicate that a relatively high garlic intake reduces the risk of developing certain cancers.

Russia - Moscow:
Scientists at the Russian Academy of Medical Sciences conducted a live double-blind placebo-controlled study on 60 type-2 diabetic patients.[8] They used time controlled garlic powder tablets and found that garlic produced a better

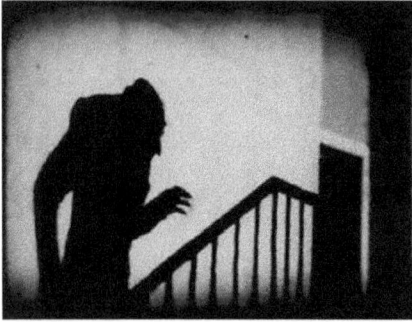

Screenshot from the 1922 Vampire film
Nosferatu, Eine Symphonie des Grauens

metabolic control in patients due to lowered blood glucose and triglyceride levels. These scientists now recommend garlic in conjunction with dietary control and other measures in the treatment of adult onset diabetes. Scientists believe the garlic helps obtain a more efficient glucose and fat metabolism, thereby contributing to the prevention of long-term complications such as heart attacks.

Singapore:

Various traditional healing traditions have long known about garlic's potent heart protective properties. A Singapore study determined that S-allylcysteine (SAC), an organosulphur-containing compound produced from garlic, is protective in myocardial infarction (heart attacks).[9]

Taiwan - Taipei:

Diallyl disulfide, a well-known component of garlic, has been demonstrated repeatedly to induce apoptosis (destruction) of many different cancer cells. Now the mechanism, according to these Taiwanese scientists, may be associated with signal transducer and activator of transcription 1 (STAT1) expression.[10]

United States - Chicago:

This study, which used a rodent experiment to examine garlic on Alzheimer's disease, concluded that aged garlic extract has a potential for preventing the progression of Alzheimer's disease.[11]

United States - New York:

In this study, scientists examined garlic's ability in preventing the infestation of the malaria parasite. Interestingly, given the extensive stories on how garlic protects against blood-suckers (vampires – 'mosquitoes'), they found that allicin, a well-known compound in garlic is also a cysteine protease inhibitor. These scientists learned that the malaria parasite uses an enzyme (cysteine protease) to manipulate its own surface protein membrane along with the protective membranes of host cells (human or other mammals) in order to gain entry. Garlic constituent allicin inhibits the parasitical protein membrane (made from circumsporozoite protein) manipulation and thereby prevents or reduces invasion in vitro and in vivo in two of the four life cycles of the parasites' sporozoites (stage of parasite when initially entering the bloodstream) and merozoits (stage of parasite when it asexually reproduces inside the red blood-cell).[12]

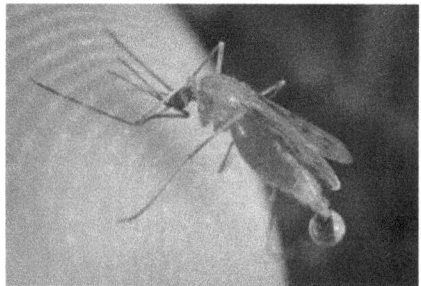

Picture of a female mosquito Anophele feeding.
Courtesy: CDC

Did you know that people with sickle cell anemia are immune to malaria? There are statistics on how many people contract malaria, statistics on how many people die of malaria; but there are no statistics on how many people who live in malaria regions never contract the disease. Why and how does the internal architecture of those differ from those who are victimized?

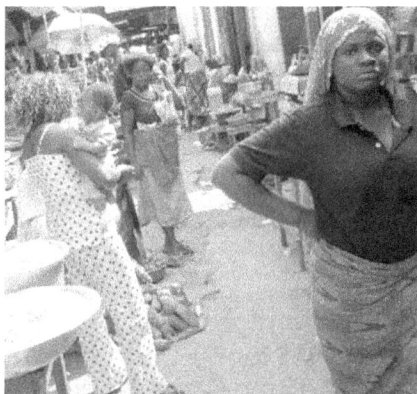

Garlic. Makola Market, Accra 2008

PREPARATIONS:
Availability: Fresh cooked garlic capsules, oils, tinctures, drops, and syrups are readily available in stores. For specific ailments, consult a knowledgeable healthcare provider. Cuban herbalists do not like to use capsules because they believe that the therapeutic chemical reaction starts in the mouth and the experience of tasting it is an extremely important part of therapy.

Internal preparation: Decoctions (a strong tea) can be made by boiling 20 grams (about three quarter ounce) of garlic in half a liter of water (about three cups) for five minutes. Keep refrigerated; it can be used safely for a day. Drink three cups a day. Do not use when pregnant or nursing. Do not give to children under ten.

Asthma: Take up to ten cloves of garlic and boil them in a cup of water, add a teaspoon of honey and drink at nighttime while hot.

Topical preparation: For topical use to heal fungal and bacterial infections, 100 grams (about four ounces) of peeled crushed garlic are placed in half a liter (about a pint) of distilled water for four days at about 40-50 degrees Fahrenheit. Shake vigorously once a day. Filter through a cheesecloth the fifth day until fluid is clear. Store at room temperature in a dark glass bottle. It may be used for up to one week. Apply topically once or twice a day to the affected area. Do not make this preparation any stronger than this concentration. Sensitive people may still find this to cause dermatitis and inflammation. Drops are used to treat ear infections.

WARNING:
Garlic, especially at high dosages, can cause skin irritation, kidney and digestive disorders. Do not use in high dose during pregnancy. Do not use if you have a scheduled surgery to avoid loss of blood from garlic's blood thinning effect.

Possible interaction with drugs:
The action of blood thinning (antiplatelet and anticoagulant) drugs or supplements such as heparin, warfarin, gingko biloba or aspirin may be further activated by the mild blood-thinning properties of garlic. This could be good thinning or harmful depending on the patient's specific condition. Consult your health care practitioner.

1 Herodotus. *The Histories of Herodotus*. Random House. New York. 1997. Second book, 125.

2 Howard EW, Ling MT, Chua CW, Cheung HW, Wang X, Wong YC. *Garlic-derived S-allylmercaptocysteine is a novel in vivo antimetastatic*

agent for androgen-independent prostate cancer. Cancer Biology Group, Department of Anatomy, Faculty of Medicine, University of Hong Kong, Hong Kong. Clin Cancer Res. 2007 Mar 15;13(6):1847-56.

3 Singh SP, Abraham SK, Kesavan PC. *Radio-protection of mice following garlic pretreatment.* School of Life Sciences, Jawaharlal Nehru Unviersity, New Delhi, India. Br J Cancer Suppl. 1996 Jul;27:S102-4.

4 Tedeschi P, Maietti A, Boggian M, Vecchiati G, Brandolini V. *Fungitoxicity of lyophilized and spray-dried garlic extracts.* Department of Pharmaceutical Science, University of Ferrara, Ferrara, Italy. J Environ Sci Health B. 2007 Sep;42(7):795-9.

5 Okada Y, Tanaka K, Sato E, Okajima H. *Kinetic and mechanistic studies of allicin as an antioxi-dant.* Department of Analytical Chemistry, Faculty of Health Sciences, Kyorin University, 476 Miyasita-cho, Hachioji, Tokyo, 192-8508, Japan. Org Biomol Chem. 2006 Nov 21;4(22):4113-7.

6 Fukao H, Yoshida H, Tazawa Y, Hada T. *Anti-thrombotic effects of odorless garlic powder both in vitro and in vivo.* Department of Nutritional Sciences, Faculty of Food Culture, Kurashiki Sakuyo University, Japan. Biosci Biotechnol Biochem. 2007 Jan;71(1):84-90.

7 Herman-Antosiewicz A, Powolny AA, Singh SV. *Molecular targets of cancer chemoprevention by garlic-derived organosulfides.* Department of Molecular Biology, University of Gdask, Kladki 24, 80-822 Gdask, Poland. Acta Pharmacol Sin. 2007 Sep;28(9):1355-1364.

8 Sobenin IA, Nedosugova LV, Filatova LV, Balabolkin MI, Gorchakova TV, Orekhov AN. *Metabolic effects of time-released garlic powder tablets in type 2 diabetes mellitus: the results of double-blinded placebo-controlled study.* Institute of General Pathology and Pathophysiology, Russian Academy of Medical Sciences, Moscow, Russia. Acta Diabetol. September 6, 2007.

9 Chuah SC, Moore PK, Zhu YZ. *S-allylcysteine mediates cardioprotection in an acute myocardi-al infarction rat model via a hydrogen sulphide mediated pathway.* Dept. of Pharmacology, National University of Singapore, Singapore, Singapore. Am J Physiol Heart Circ Physiol. August 31, 2007

10 Lu HF, Yang JS, Lin YT, Tan TW, Ip SW, Li YC, Tsou MF, Chung JG. *Diallyl Disulfide Induced Signal Transducer and Activator of Transcription 1 Expression in Human Colon Cancer Colo 205 Cells using Differential Display RT-PCR y.* Department of Clinical Pathology, Cheng Hsin Rehabilitation Medical Center, Tai-pei, Taiwan, R.O.C. Cancer Genomics Proteom-ics. 2007 Mar-Apr;4(2):93-8.

11 Chauhan NB, Sandoval J. Amelioration of early cognitive deficits by *aged garlic extract in Alzheimer's transgenic mice.* Research and Development (151), Jesse Brown VA Medical Center Chicago, Department of Anesthesiology, University of Illinois at Chicago, IL 60612, USA. Phytother Res. 2007 Jul;21(7):629-40.

12 Coppi A, Cabinian M, Mirelman D, Sinnis P. *Antimalarial activity of allicin, a biologically active compound from garlic cloves.* Department of Medical Parasitology, New York University School of Medicine, 341 East 25th Street, New York, NY 10010, USA.

Amharic: Nechshingurt
Dutch: Knoflook
French: Ail cultivé
German: Knoblauch
Hebrew: Shum
Hindi: Lasun
Homeopathic: Allium sativum
(All-s.)
Italian: Aglio comune
Korean: Kallik
Latin: Allium sativum
Russian: Chesnok
Sanskrit: Lashuna
Spanish: Ajo
Swahili: Kitunguu samu
Tigrinya: Sa da shgurti
Twi: Gyene kankan

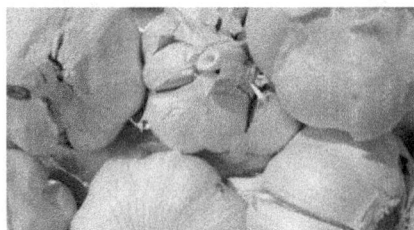

Growth: Garlic is an annual plan that is available as hundreds of species ranging between 1 – 4 feet in height. Bulb grows below ground.

Native to: Mediterranean and Central Asia but today is grown pretty much anywhere.

How to grow garlic: Garlic plants are very easy to grow in pots and gardens alike. The individual garlic clove is the seed. Plant them upright with the pointy end up and the 'flat' end down, about an inch deep into moist and good organic soil. Each garlic clove will produce a bulb containing about a couple dozen cloves themselves. With that in mind space them about 3-4 inches apart to avoid crowding.

Time to seed: To grow big and savory bulbs with potent medicinal properties may take a bit of experience. It starts with choosing a potent and rich clove stock. Pick the best from your last season or buy good stock from a trusted local organic grocer or farmer. Break the bulb just prior to planting to separate the individual cloves. Use only those cloves that come of the base easily and cleanly.

Garlic can be planted in late fall or early spring. The fall and spring equinoxes in either the northern or southern hemisphere are generally a good marker to plant garlic. Garlic planted late in the year will develop roots first and may develop a short top shoot which will quickly grow after the last frost of the year in spring has vanished. While garlic can handle some frost and winter condition it is advised to cover the winter garlic with a layer of straw/ mulch for extreme frost protection and for moisture retention later. However, if you want to grow garlic in a warmer climate you need to cool the garlic to about 50° F for 2 to 3 week to trigger the impulse to sprout.

Sun: Full sun.

Zone: Garlic is very hardy in zones 7 – 10. However, garlic lovers all over the world have success stories attesting to the fact that all zones can support the growth of garlic. Some species will do better than others under the many various climate conditions. Ask a local grower who has some good experience and try to replicate method and species.

Soil: Rich, organic well drained soil. Use natural manure to fertilize the soil to enhance chances of growing potent bulbs. Keep weeds at bay. Keep the early garlic evenly moist but not wet. Once the plant is established an occasional watering is enough especially if you use mulch. Reduce watering to near zero a few weeks before harvest time. This may take some practice and experience.

Harvest: Rule of thumb, when about half of the lengths of the leaves of the plant has turned brown and begins to wither away it is time to harvest. Double-check to see if the bulb is large and full and without cracks. Small bulbs – too early;

cracked bulbs – too late.

Pull the bulbs with the help of a small shovel and gently remove most of the soil without bruising the bulbs. Gently braid them together by their shoots not unlike in the old vampire moves where garlic braids are used for protection. Hang them in a dark and dry place, at about room temperature, with even and gentle ventilation, for a two to three weeks until they are evenly dry. Look for dry 'wrappers' but bulbs fat and rich with nutrients.

Now it is time to select those great bulbs for your next harvest and just put them aside as they are. Keep the in a dark and dry place until it is time to plant them.

The rest of the garlic bulbs must now be readied for storage or consumption. For eating cut the roots, leaving about ½ an inch in place and cut the top leaves without damaging the deeper protective wrappers. This keeps them fresh. Remove the dry dirt and the dirty outer layer of the wrappers and place the bulbs into a net, which you can hang into your pantry or kitchen area for easy access.

Attracts friends: Garlic not just protects against 'vampires' but also serves as a garden pest deterrent and is often planted at the boarders of other crops more prone to succumb to fungi other garden pests.

Environmental benefits: Protects some large leaf vegetables from aphids and snails such as cabbage and lettuce. Deters Japanese beetle.

Storage: In cool, dry and well-ventilated place garlic can last for up to a year. Store only undamaged bulbs and cloves. Remember to not to put the garlic bulbs or cloves into a refrigerator or as soon you take them out and expose the garlic to room temperature it will be initiated to sprout, making it unsuitable for cooking and consumption.

ZINGIBER
OFFICINALE

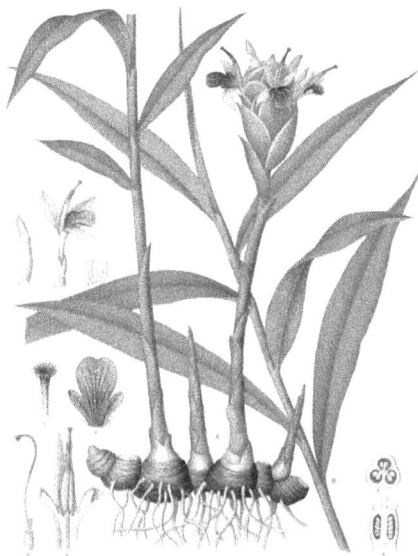

Köhler's Medicinal Plants 1887

Ginger

Trust given
appropriately
will melt away
all fears, anxi-
eties and even
dread.

Once upon a time, a country is tortured by famine and poverty. Two innocent children are taken deep into the woods and abandoned by their parents. An old woman practicing cannibalism uses a beautiful and rich-smelling gingerbread house to lure these children inside. By the end of the tale, the witch is dead, and the kids have an abandon of gingerbread signaling the dawn of better days to come.

The Grimm Brothers took the famous fairy tale of Hänsel and Gretel and transformed it into written word. Even in those olden days of Germany the 'fairy tale' properties of ginger were to entice, seduce, provide abandon, and ultimately contribute to freedom from the nauseating anxiety born in the swamps of poverty and in the fears for survival.

Ginger is now grown all over the tropical and

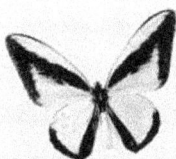

I grow just below the surface on the edge of your reality. I am grounded above and below and seduce both worlds into feeling safe. I embrace new experiences and I trust that life is good and true and beautiful. When your senses edge up against mine perhaps you too can feel safe and trust life but a bit more each time.

subtropical world. However, this was not always so. It is thought that ginger famous for its warm tasting, refreshing and strong scented rhizome, the subterranean, horizontally growing part of the plant which is often mistaken for its root, originated in the south-eastern part of the Asian continent. Ginger has been used effectively as a medicinal plant for thousands of years. It is indispensable to Chinese, Arabic (Unani - Tibbs) and Indian (Ayurvedic) traditional medicine and has a solid health and safety record when used appropriately. But what is the connection between the fairy tale and medicine?

Parts used: Rhizome

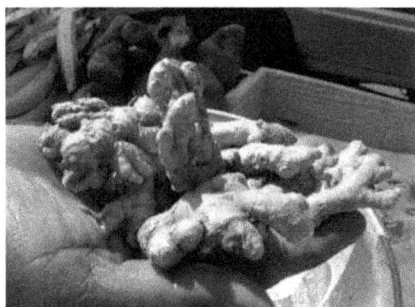

Global summary:
Used to treat: Coughs, colds, bronchitis, nausea (from chemotherapy and surgery, travel sickness, sea sickness or morning sickness) and dyspeptic problems, stomach ulcers, spasms, arthritis, muscle sprains and generalized weakness, high cholesterol and loss of appetite. It is used to treat menstrual cramps and is valued as an aphrodisiac due to its generally stimulating effects. Ginger is known to help in cases of heart disease where damaging clotting and atherosclerosis (plaque lined arteries) are present and can function to tone and strengthen your whole system.

Used as a(n): Antitussive (cough suppressant) and expectorant (helps to bring up phlegm), antibacterial, anti-emetic (suppresses nausea), antispasmodic decreases cramps), carminative (decreases flatulence/gas), stimulates digestive juices, anti-ulcer, tonic (restores normal tone/function; revitalizing), anti-arthritic, anti-inflammatory, anti-oxidant, blood thinner, anti tumor, cancer preventative.

Cuba's traditional uses:
In Cuba, Ginger belongs to the realm of Oggun and is used for the treatment of menstrual pains and nausea.

Summary medicinal uses and properties supported by scientific studies:
Anti-emetic (morning sickness, sea sickness, post surgery sickness), analgesic, anti-inflammatory, anti-oxidant, antibacterial (Helicobacter pylori), cardio tonic, may enhance sperm motility and count, stomach ulcer preventative, hepaprotective, DNA protective, and may be protective against various breast cancer lines in vitro. Ginger may also be useful in treating certain diabetic conditions due to its ability to lower serum glucose, cholesterol and triacylglycerol levels.

Austria - Graz:
These researchers point out that while the properties of ginger and cannabis in the reduction of nausea and vomiting are well established by a series of scientific studies, the focus on special receptor sites involved in producing the very nausea and vomiting is still not very well understood and more research is suggested.[1]

China - Jinan:
Components of ginger have been found

to protect the epithelium (tissue lining inside the arteries) when exposed to an environment of high fat diets. This rodent based study confirmed that ginger was able to reduce the thickening of the artery wall as measured by intima-media thickness of the aorta.[2]

German Commission E:
Approved for the treatment of: "Dyspepsia, prevention of motion sickness."

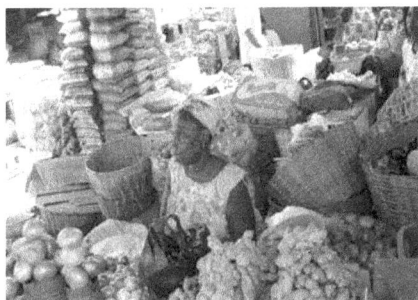

Ginger. Makola Market, Accra 2008.

India - Mysore:
According to this study and echoing an allopathic consensus, physical conditions that can produce an environment conducive to ulcer formations are the presence of Helicobacter pylori, the bacteria involved in ulcer production, oxidative stress, stomach irritability (due to increased gastric cell proton potassium ATPase activity (PPA) or perturbation of mucosal defense) and nonsteroidal anti-inflammatory drugs (NSAID's) such as vioxx, ibuprofen, aspirin or naproxen.

These Indian scientists determined that ginger protects the body from stomach ulcer formation by multiple means: inhibiting Helicobacter pylori, exhibits ability to scavenge free radicals (strong anti-oxidant), inhibiting lipid peroxidation and by displaying DNA protection. The study concludes that ginger may be an inexpensive and multi-pronged approach to protect against stomach ulcer formation.[3]

Kuwait - Safat:
The effectiveness of ginger to alleviate the difficulties of diabetic rats to breakdown sugar and convert it to usable energy was examined in this study, which discovered that ginger at 500mg/kg was able to lower blood glucose, cholesterol and triacylglycerol levels when compared to the control group of rats not receiving the treatment.[4]

Saudi Arabia - Riyadh:
Ginger has long been in Unani traditional medicine to enhance sexual function in males. Scientists used a rodent experiment to test the influence of ginger as part of their diet. The results showed that ginger significantly increased sperm motility (movement) and content without any toxic side effects.[5]

South Africa - Durban:
This researcher supports the time-proven use of ginger by traditional African healers as an effective means to treat painful and chronic arthritic inflammatory conditions and its use to achieve better metabolic control in patients with type-2 adult-onset diabetes.[6]

South Korea - Seoul:
Ginger, a spice commonly used in Korean traditional medicine and cuisine, has been proven by researchers to have the ability to protect and strengthen the heart and liver, function as an anti-inflammatory and now has been examined with regards to its potential to inhibit breast cancer cell growth.[7]

Switzerland - Zürich:
In this study, thousands of volunteers,

participated to determine how well seven different commonly used prophylactic of seasickness worked. The data was gathered during whale watching tours in Norway. In the control group, not receiving any prophylactic, 80% showed signs of seasickness, namely nausea with vomiting and malaise. In the group receiving a prophylactic amongst seven various agents, only about 4 – 10% of the individuals experienced nausea with vomiting; about 16 – 23% experienced malaise independent of which prophylactic they took, thus indicating a similar effectiveness in preventing seasickness. The agents were: ginger root, cinnarizine, cinnarizine with domperidone, cyclizine, dimenhydrinate with caffeine, meclozine with caffeine, and scopolamine, which seemed the least effective.[8]

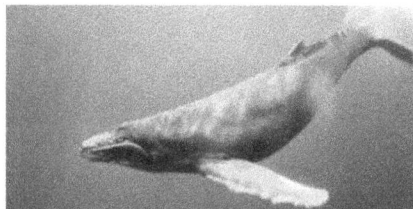

Humpback Whale. Courtesy: National Oceanic and Atmospheric Administration

Thailand – Bangkok:
In this double-blind placebo controlled study ginger has proven to be effective in preventing nausea and vomiting associated with female patients receiving major gynecological surgery. The patients in the treatment group received two capsules of ginger taken one hour before the procedure (one capsule containing 0.5 gram of ginger powder).[9]

Thailand – Bangkok:
Another study discovered that 650mg of ginger given three times daily for a total of 4 days to pregnant women experiencing morning sickness worked even better than vitamin B-6 (another commonly used natural supplement to reduce nausea and vomiting during early pregnancies).[10]

PREPARATIONS:
Infusion preparation: Pour a cup of boiling water over one teaspoon of chopped fresh root and let sit for ten minutes.

Decoction preparation: For topical use on sprains, pour a cup of cold water over two tablespoons of chopped ginger, bring it to a boil, let cool to a warm temperature and apply.

Herb: Take about five gram daily to reduce swelling and pain during an arthritis flare up.

Unwanted Effects:
High doses of ginger may cause gastrointestinal and urinary irritation. Due to its ability to stimulate digestive juices it should be used with caution in cases of gallbladder stones.

WARNING:
As low doses of ginger help with morning sickness, high doses may cause abortions. For the treatment of morning sickness use no more than one gram of ginger just to be sure. Chinese doctors are using doses of over 20 grams to bring about menstruation in some female patients who have stopped menstruating without having reached menopause. At this dose ginger may cause an abortions.

Possible interaction with drugs:
Ginger has mild blood thinning properties and caution should be exercised if you are using other substances with similar properties such as aspirin, salicylic acid, warfarin, and heparin or gingko biloba.

1 Crockett SL, Schühly W, Bauer R. *Pflanzliche antiemetika. Inhaltsstoffe, molekulare wirkmechanismen und klinische evidenz.* Bereich Pharmakognosie, Institut für Pharmazeutische Wissenschaften, Universitätsplatz 4/1, Karl-Franzens-Universität Graz, A-8010 Graz, Osterreich. Pharm Unserer Zeit. 2007;36(5):381-8.

2 Wu CX, Wei XB, Ding H, Sun X, Cheng XM. *Protective effect of effective parts of Zingiber Offecinal on vascular endothelium of the experimental hyperlipidemic rats.* Department of Pharmacology, School of Medicine Shandong University, Jinan 250012, China. wcxzzl@eyou. com Zhong Yao Cai. 2006 Aug;29(8):810-3.

Amharic: Zinjibil
Dutch: Gember
French: Gingembre
German: Ingwer
Hebrew: Sangvil
Hindi: Adi
Homeopathic: Zingiber officinale
(Zing.)
Italian: Zenzevero
Korean: Jinjeo
Latin: Zingiber officinale
Russian: Imbir
Sanskrit: Shringavera
Spanish: Jengibre
Swahili: Tangawizi
Tigrinya: Jingeble
Twi: Akakaduru

3 Siddaraju MN, Dharmesh SM. Inhibition of gastric H+, K+-ATPase and Helicobacter pylori growth by phenolic antioxidants of Zingiber officinale. Department of Biochemistry and Nutrition, Central Food Technological Research Institute, Mysore 570-020, Karnataka, India. Mol Nutr Food Res. 2007 Mar;51(3):324-32.

4 Al-Amin ZM, Thomson M, Al-Qattan KK, Peltonen-Shalaby R, Ali M. *Anti-diabetic and hypolipidaemic properties of ginger (Zingiber officinale) in streptozotocin-induced diabetic rats.* Department of Biological Sciences, Faculty of Science, Kuwait University, 13060-Safat, Kuwait. Br J Nutr. 2006 Oct;96(4):660-6.

5 Qureshi S, Shah AH, Tariq M, Ageel AM. *Studies on herbal aphrodisiacs used in Arab system of medicine.* Research Centre, College of Pharmacy, King Saud University, Riyadh, Saudi Arabia. Am J Chin Med. 1989;17(1-2):57-63.

6 Ojewole JA. *Analgesic, antiinflammatory and hypoglycaemic effects of ethanol extract of Zingiber officinale (Roscoe) rhizomes (Zingiberaceae) in mice and rats.* Department of Pharmacology, Faculty of Health Sciences, University of KwaZulu-Natal, Private Bag X54001, Durban, South Africa. ojewolej@ukzn.ac.za Phytother Res. 2006 Sep;20(9):764-72.

7 Lee HS, Seo EY, Kang NE, Kim WK. [6]-*Gingerol inhibits metastasis of MDA-MB-231 human breast cancer cells.* Department of Sports Sciences, Seoul Sports Graduate University, Seoul 150-034, South Korea. J Nutr Biochem. 2007 Jul 31.

8 Schmid R, Schick T, Steffen R, Tschopp A, Wilk T. *Comparison of Seven Commonly Used Agents for Prophylaxis of Seasickness.* Institute of Social and Preventive Medicine of the University of Zurich, Switzerland. J Travel Med. 1994 Dec 1;1(4):203-206.

9 Nanthakomon T, Pongrojpaw D. *The efficacy of ginger in prevention of postoperative nausea and vomiting after major gynecologic surgery.* Department of Obstetrics and Gyecology, Faculty of Medicine, Thammasat University, Bangkok 12120, Thailand. J Med Assoc Thai. 2006 Oct;89 Suppl 4:S130-6.

10 Chittumma P, Kaewkiattikun K, Wiriyasiriwach B. *Comparison of the effectiveness of ginger and vitamin B6 for treatment of nausea and vomiting in early pregnancy: a randomized double-blind controlled trial.* Department of Obstetrics and Gynecology, Bangkok Metropolitan Administration Medical College and Vajira Hospital, Dusit, Bangkok, Thailand. J Med Assoc Thai. 2007 Jan;90(1):15-20.

Growth: Ginger is a tropical and sub-tropical perennial plant between 2 – 6 feet in height depending on which of the many species you plant.

Native to: Ginger is thought to have originated in part of Asia but is now at home in India, West Africa and the Caribbean.

How to grow ginger: Buy the type of organic ginger rhizome from a grocer you would like to grow. Look for fat, solid, robust and smooth surfaces with many buds and avoid those with cracks or a dry and wrinkled surface. Soak the rhizomes in warm water over night. Place the ginger into the planting container with the buds pointing up. Cover them with soil leaving but the surface exposed. Water the rhizomes lightly to keep them slightly moist but not wet. Once the shoots appear, after about 10 days to 2 weeks, water a bit more. During its growth cycle the plant will reach an average height of 4 feet depending on species. Most ginger species flower from July through September and some have striking foliage.

If you want to keep ginger in a pot use 3 – 5 gallon containers to allow the plant to expand nicely.

Time to plant: While it is more common in tropical and sub-tropical climates ginger can be grown outdoors anywhere where the climate can sustain its growth. If not, Ginger can be grown inside in pots. Keep the plant inside until you can be reasonably sure that the average outdoor temperature will be about 75º F. Once the temperature goes below 50º F and approach near freezing the plant will die. Ginger is very frost sensitive. For outside planting choose a wind-sheltered location.

Sun: Young plants need a bright spot but must be protected by shade. Even once the plant is established shade or at least a majority of partial shade is crucial for many ginger species to thrive.

Zone: 9 – 11

Soil: Organic well drained potting soil enriched with compost. Ginger can be grown in many different soil environments. If growing in containers place some rock at the bottom of the pot to avoid over watering.

Harvest: While in general your sign to indicate the proper time to harvest is when the leafs begin to turn brown and wilt away, most plants grow fast enough that parts can be used after only about 4 – 6 months of growth. Once the plant is established and growing well, cut some of the new vertical shoots, as you need them for cooking of medicine. To harvest the rhizome cut the new horizontally growing rhizomes off the base-rhizome of the plant. Clean the rhizomes gently and place the on a clean and breathable cover in the sun to dry.

To know the variation of specific tastes and special medicinal properties takes knowledge and experience and is a 'science' by itself. However, the general properties discussed in this book are applicable to most species of ginger. There are a great many books available on how to work with ginger much more precisely and specifically.

Ginger goes dormant in colder winters. It 'hibernates.' Let it dry and begin care with the new cycle of spring.

Attracts friends: Some ginger flowers give of a spice scent that attracts bees, butterflies and birds.

Environmental benefits: The spice scent of the plant repels some garden pest.

Storage: Fresh ginger can be stored safely for a few weeks when kept in a brown paper bag and placed in the refrigerator. Store dry powdered ginger in a tight container and keep in a dark and dry place.

Aframomum melegueta. Limbe, Cameroon

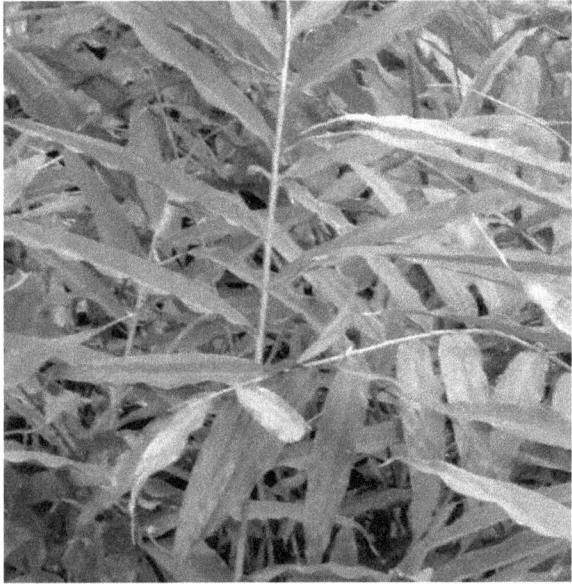

Grains of Paradise

One grain of sand can give life to a whole universe, one grain of care can give life to so much more.

Grains of paradise, such wondrous allure embedded in a name, perhaps finds its origin in legend long forgotten. However, this spice's name echoes with healing meaning to the many people recovering from broken and dislocated bones at the Aponche Memorial Herbal Clinic in Accra, Ghana.

The clinic, specializing in traditional bonesetting, uses grains of paradise (also known as wisa) in a topical paste applied to fractures. It speeds the healing process and acts as an antiseptic to prevent infections. I had heard about traditional bonesetters from a few Nigerian studies, which suggested a possible marriage, or at least love affair, between orthopedic surgeons and traditional bonesetters based on an interesting observation. Every orthopedic doctor comes

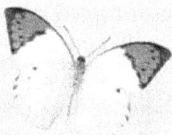

My names carry the whispers of deeper meaning; 'grains of paradise' the living echo of a heavenly sound, a divine color that emanates from the act of turning guilt and its belief in punishment into an appropriate release of anger, forgiveness and a positive change. Alligator pepper; a reminder that you are the sovereign author of your world, go write a life without fear; instead create a life filled with adventure and deep mystery.

across a fracture that will not take. Some of these were taken to a bonesetter who managed to succeed where the medical doctor had not.[1] Respectively, the Nigerian researchers also noted that some infection experienced in a traditional bonesetting could benefit from 'modern' infection control measures.[2] So, when I heard about the reputation of the Aponche clinic and its use of spices and herbs to speed bone healing and prevent infections, I wanted to see for myself.

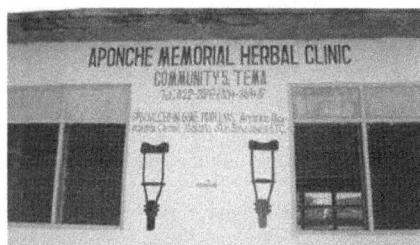

After obtaining permission from the Ministry of Health, I visited the clinic and interviewed everyone recovering in the male ward. I took their accident histories, inspected the fracture sites and checked extremities for any signs of infection. I found none. All reset fractures were in natural alignment with no loss of sensation or signs of diminished perfusion. The patients were comfortable and all recounted a similar story. Before the fractured bones were set at the clinic the patients were given a plant preparation to drink for pain control.

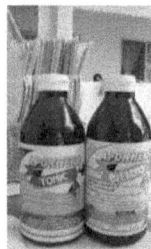

Aponche non-narcotic herbal analgesic.

Setting a broken bone in a conscious patient is normally a very painful process. I know, because I have done it myself many times during my service at the San Francisco Department of Health. Yet, my experience included the benefit of strong, injectable narcotics for the patients, though, still to often agonizing screams.

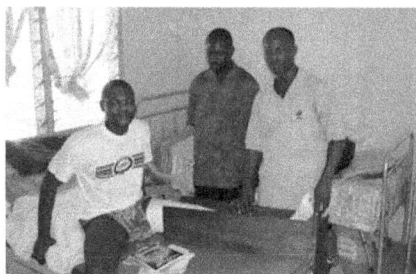

Aponche Bonesetters, Paul Ntima and Samuel Essilfie. Accra, Ghana 2008

Here, however, the patients all reported an ability to cope with the pain, or in fact went to sleep during or shortly after the reduction of the fracture. This was the first time I had heard of a natural substance void of the presence of a narcotic.

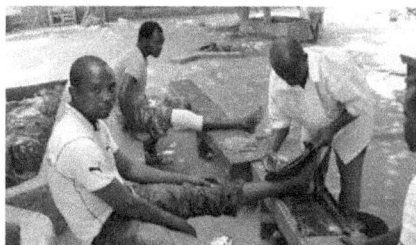

Grains of paradise containing topical paste.

The plant's ability to promote wound healing has not gone unnoticed by the pharmaceutical industry and academia. An article in the Washington Post reported on research conducted at Rutgers University's Biotechnology Center.[3] The center apparently found an active component in grains of paradise that acts as a strong anti-inflammatory. The article suggests that the pharmaceutical companies have high hopes that it could fill the void left by the 'killer-anti-inflammatory drugs' Vioxx and Co.

Parts used: All parts (Fruit, flower, seed, root, shoots, leaves)

Global summary:
Used to treat: Bone fractures, pain, fever, cholera, constipation, venom injuries, cancer, tumors, skin infections (measles, fungus, leprosy, yaws-tropical bacterial infection of skin/bones, inflammation), malaria, decreased libido in males and females, infertility, excessive bleeding after birth, balancing lactation, bleeding wounds, schistosomiasis and stomach ulcers.

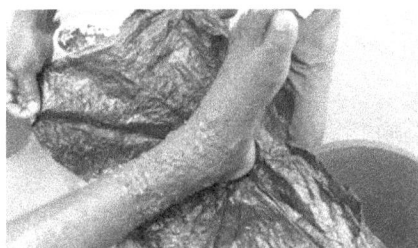

Used as a(n): aphrodisiac, antidote (poisonous bites from insects or snakes), lung tonic, anti-microbial (viral, bacterial, fungal and certain parasites) and as an agent to promote healing of bone injuries, anti-inflammatory, bleeding, and gastro-intestinal difficulties.

Summary medicinal uses and properties supported by scientific studies:
Promoting wound healing by cell membrane support, anti-oxidant, and analgesic when inflammation present, molluscicidal, anti-diarrhea, anti-microbial, may enhance sexual interest and function.

Cameroon – Buea:
Scientists tested several African plants' abilities to rid bodies of water of their snail population.[4] The spice proved highly capable of ridding the waterways of snails carrying parasites

such as schistosomiasis.

Cameroon – Yaoundé:
Researchers, using a rodent model, discovered that 115mg/kg of a water-based extract of grains of paradise significantly increased male arousal and sexual function.[5]

Ghana – Kumasi:
This study offers an overview of several local Ghanaian herbs and spices,[6] which have been known traditionally to exhibit anti-microbial properties. Results reaffirm the age-old practice of using grains of paradise for wound healing.

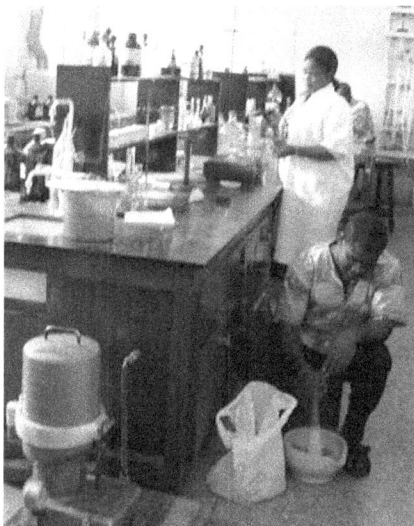

Centre for Scientific Research into Plant Medicine. Mampong, Ghana. 2008

Holland – Wageningen:
Dutch scientists looked at a variety of medicinal plants used by hunters on the island of Trinidad. Hunters used grains of paradise for themselves and their dogs[7] as part of the traditional Trinidadian treatment repertoire in addressing wounds and venomous bites (scorpions or snakes).

Nigeria - Lagos:

Water-based extracts made from seeds of grains of paradise were found to have a significant ability to reduce diarrhea. In addition, they appeared to possess inhibitive actions on prostaglandins (hormone like fatty acids) productions[8].

Nigeria - Lagos:

Rodents receiving 100-500mg of the water-based extract of the spice experienced a significant reduction of castor oil-induced diarrhea.[9]

Nigeria - Ibadan:

Scientists discovered several potential observable explanations for the usage of the spice in age-old wound healing practices. The spice has the ability to stabilize the cell membrane[10] of injured tissue sites thus possibly reducing the need and speed for reconstruction. Furthermore, it has also been noted to have strong anti-oxidant properties enabling the body to more effectively scavenge free radicals common in injuries.

Nigeria - Ibadan:

Another study from the same university shows that the analgesic (pain reducing) properties of the spice are specific to sites with inflamed tissue only. They do not reduce the pain perceptions of non-inflamed tissue sites.[11]

PREPARATIONS:

Traditional healers around Mt. Cameroon have used the plant leaves in inhalation steam treatments to reduce the symptoms of respiratory ailments due to colds, coughs and flu. In addition, the leaves deliver relief through respiration to patients suffering from malaria.

Root decoctions are used in West Africa to reduce excessive lactation in new mothers and to treat excessive bleeding after giving birth.

Fresh fruit are used to enhance sexual stimulation and sensation in males and females.

The seeds are used to improve male sexual function. Try 250mg to 1gm of the seeds an hour before sexual contact or a range of 2.5 mg/kg - 10mg/kg twice a day to achieve results. The aframomum family consists of dozens of subspecies; and aframomum stipulatum has been noted to especially improve penile rigidity and endurance.

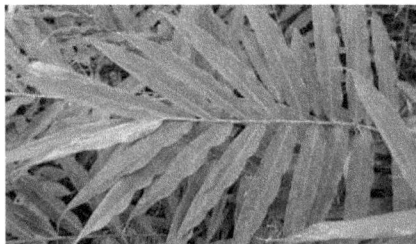

Fresh leafs of Grains of Paradise. Limbe, Cameroon 2008

Unwanted Effects:
Nigeria - Uturu:

This investigation suggested a possibly mild and transient side-effect of blurred vision.[12]

Possible interaction with drugs:

The spice may inhibit prostaglandins (fatty acids that act like hormones). Prostaglandins are involved in a variety of biological functions: control parts of digestion, expansion or constriction of smooth muscles affecting blood pressure and respiration, platelet homeostasis, inflammatory reactions, hormone production and more. Several prostaglandins products such as Caverject are sold to treat erectile dysfunction in males. Is this spice a more natural way to achieve virility?

1 Omonzejele F. Peter. *Current Ethical and other Problems in the Practice of African Traditional Medicine.* Department of Philosophy, University of Benin, Benin City, Nigeria.

2 JE Onuminya. *The role of the traditional bonesetter in primary fracture care in Nigeria.* Department of Orthopaedics and Traumatology, Faculty of Clinical Sciences, College of Medicine, Ambrose Alli University, PMB 14, Ekpoma, Edo State, Nigeria. S Afr Med J 2004; 94: 652-658.

3 Cheryl Lyn Dybas. *Gorilla Staple Adds Spice to New Drugs.* The Washington Post, Monday, November 27, 2006; Page A8

4 Ndamukong KJ, Ntonifor NN, Mbuh J, Atemnkeng AF, Akam MT. *Molluscicidal activity of some Cameroonian plants on Bulinus species.* Department of Administrative Affairs, University of Buea, Cameroon. East Afr Med J. 2006 Mar;83(3):102-9.

5 Kamtchouing P, Mbongue GY, Dimo T, Watcho P, Jatsa HB, Sokeng SD. *Effects of Aframomum melegueta and Piper guineense on sexual behaviour of male rats.* Laboratoire de Physiologie Animale, Faculté des Sciences, Université de Yaoundé I, Yaoundé, Cameroun. mbongue@yahoo.com Behav Pharmacol. 2002 May;13(3):243-7.

6 Konning GH, Agyare C, Ennison B. *Antimicrobial activity of some medicinal plants from Ghana.* Department of Pharmaceutics, Faculty of Pharmacy, Kwame Nkrumah University of Science and Technology, Kumasi, Ghana. Fitoterapia. 2004 Jan;75(1):65-7

7 Lans C, Harper T, Georges K, Bridgewater E. *Medicinal and ethnoveterinary remedies of hunters in Trinidad.* Group Technology and Agrarian Development, Hollandseweg 1, 6706 KN Wageningen University, the Netherlands. Cher2lans@netscape.net BMC Complement Altern Med. 2001;1:10.

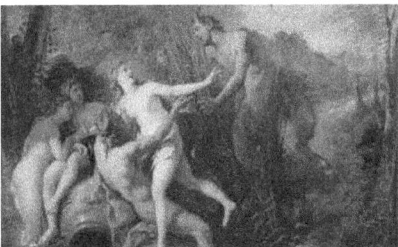

Alluring Pan and Syrinx. Courtesy: Jean-François de Troy. (1679-1752)

Amharic: Kewrerima
Ashanti: Apokua
Dutch: Paradijszaad
Ewe: Awusa
French: Graines de paradis
German: Paradieskörner
Hebrew: Garger gan ha-eden
Italian: Grani del paradiso
Korean: Meligueta
Latin: Aframomum melegueta
Russian: Rajskiye zyorna
Spanish: Malagueta
Tigrinya: Korerima
Twi: Wisa

8 Umukoro, S., Ashorobi, R. B. *Pharmacological evaluation of the antidiarrhoeal activity of Aframomum melegueta seed extract.* Department of Pharmacology, College of Medicine, University of Lagos, P.M.B. 12003, Lagos, Nigeria. West African Journal of Pharmacology and Drug Research, 2004, (Vol. 19).

9 Umukoro, S., Ashorobi, R. B. *Effect of Aframomum melegueta seed extract on castor oil-induced diarrhea.* Department of Pharmacology, College of Medicine, University of Lagos, Nigeria. Pharmaceutical biology (Pharm. biol.) ISSN 1388-0209 2005, vol. 43, no4, pp. 330-333 [4 page(s) (article)] (17 ref.)

10 Umukoro S, Ashorobi BR. *Further pharmacological studies on aqueous seed extract of Aframomum melegueta in rats.* Department of Pharmacology and Therapeutics, College of Medicine, University of Ibadan, Nigeria. J Ethnopharmacol. 2008 Feb 12;115(3):489-93.

11 Umukoro S, Ashorobi RB. *Further studies on the antinociceptive action of aqueous seed extract of Aframomum melegueta.* Department of Pharmacology and Thera peutics, University of Ibadan, Ibadan, Nigeria. umusolo@yahoo.com J Ethnopharmacol. 2007 Feb 12;109(3):501-4.

12 Igwe SA, Emeruwa IC, Modie JA. *Ocular toxicity of Afromomum melegueta (alligator pepper) on healthy Igbos of Nigeria.* Department of Pharmacology and Therapeutics, College of Medicine and Health Sciences, Abia State University, Uturu, Nigeria. J Ethnopharmacol. 1999 Jun;65(3):203-6.

Growth: Grains of Paradise is a perennial up to 3 feet in height and similar in look and growth to ginger or turmeric.

Native to: Native to West Africa but grows also is other regions on the continent.

How to grow grains of paradise: The plant is grown from seed. One seedpod can contain hundred of small seeds.

Time to seed: Year around.

Sun: Partial shade.

Zone: 11-12. Average coolest temperature in coastal Ghana is about 24°C.

Soil: Rich, well drained soil.

Harvest: The fresh seedpods are harvested when they turn to a dark red coloration. To dry them, place them as a single layer, in the sun on a breathable, clean surface for about a week to ten days. The pods are dry when the have a wrinkled, black appearance and are hard and solid when you touch them.

Attracts friends: The lily-like flower attracts bees and butterflies.

Environmental benefits: This plant can easily be grown in local West African gardens on small lots of land and produce enough seeds to supplement the household income of the grower's families. The plant will mature in less than a year and can produce seeds for ten or more years.

Storage: The dried pods containing hundreds of seeds 'for safe keeping' can be stored for a long time as long as it is in a dry and dark place. Break the pods and use the loose seeds as needed. Grind the seeds into a fine powder. Any unbroken seed pieces will crunch like sand when you chew on them making the experience somewhat unpleasant.

COMMIPHORA
MYRRHA

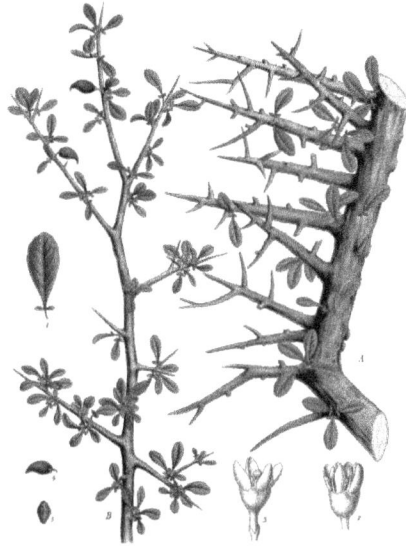

Köhler's Medicinal Plants 1887

Myrrh

Touch me with
fire - and I will
bloom into a
mist that can
transcend the
separations of
heaven and
earth.

Myrrh, an essential element in the complex embalming process of mummification, is perhaps older than the bible. 'It is said that a sacred bird, one of a kind, similar in size and shape of an eagle but covered in red and golden plumage lived in the lands of Arabia for five hundred years. Upon the death of the parent the newborn Phoenix would make a sphere of myrrh. Into the sphere s/he would place the dead parental body and s/he would carry it such into the ancient land of Egypt, to the Temple of the Sun, to bury it.'[1]

Somehow, myrrh held not just importance to the legendary phoenix, but to priests, monarchs, pharaohs and merchants all long the ancient spice routes. It is mentioned in the 3,600 years old Ebers papyrus as a remedy for diarrhea, toothaches and sore throats.

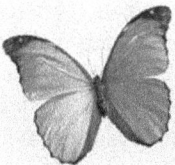

Like my branches, my scent reaches upwards to the sky; like my roots my scent is firmly grounded in the earth. I know where I begin and where I end. I am here, I am gentle and I am strong. Reach high into the sky and deep into the earth – and with great care, nourish yourself, take back what rightfully belongs to you – your power. Dream a dream against the evening sky cloaked in the deep and satisfying safety of the earth. Myrrhhhhhhhh.

An age-old Greek myth tells the story of Myrrha who was the daughter of an ancient king of Cyprus. According to the myth Myrrha is punished with lust for her father. This was not for her 'sins' but for the 'sin' of her mother for claiming Myrrha was more beautiful than the Goddess of love, Aphrodite. In her lust for her father, Myrrha, disguises herself as a prostitute, seduces her father and gets pregnant. When her father finds out he tries to kill her. Myrrha prays to the gods to turn her into a tree so her father cannot kill her. The gods comply. She is turned into a tree and manages to give birth to her son, Adonis, conceived by her father. As fate would have it this ancient soap opera of incest, codependency and victimhood further unfolds with Aphrodite falling for Adonis the extraordinarily handsome fruit of Myrrha.

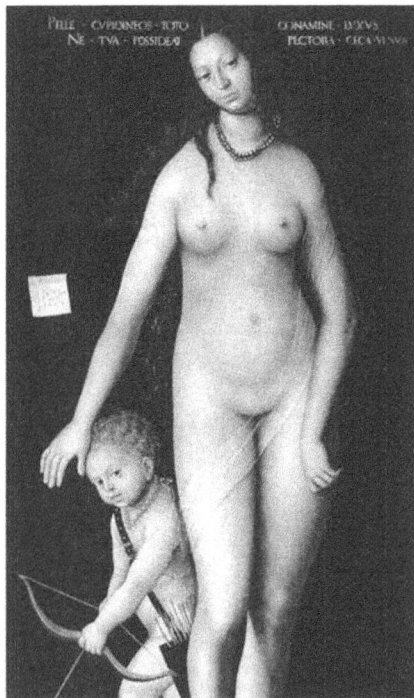

Venus and Cupid. Lucas Cranach der Ältere. Germany 1509

Perhaps this legend can speak to why myrrh is a common ingredient in many skin beautification products?

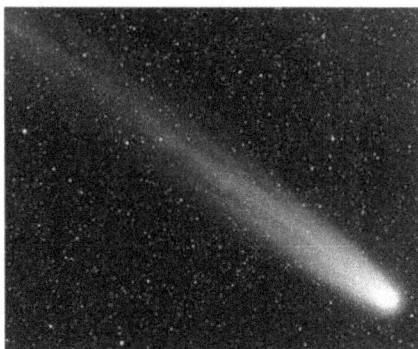

'Bearded' Comet. Courtesy: NASA

Myrrh was burned in ancient times as incense as it is today. Like a comet's veil pours through the velvet night, myrrh resign, once touched by fire, also blooms like a whispy veil towards the sky. Both intertwined as age-old symbols for extreme longevity, death, and a connection to the afterlife.

The ancients were well informed about its ability to produce certain thoughts after emotional and psychological states. It was essential for funerals, for meditation and as medicine. Myrrh apparently originated in the land of Punt, now the area of Ethiopia, Eritrea, Djibouti and Somalia, where its smoke is used also to keep snakes away. Myrrh is dried tree sap from the Commiphora, a tree of many closely related species that does well in such extreme climates as that of the high and dry parts of East Africa.

Myrrh contains several different chemically active compounds belonging to the functional group Alkenes. Bacteria cannot grow on myrrh, which might explain why it is an ingredient for funerals and mouthwash, and why it is used in different traditional medicine as a treatment for wounds and inflammations. Myrrh has been used in Ayurvedic, Unani, and Chinese traditional medicines for centuries.

An Egyptian company has begun marketing myrrh under the name of Mirazid. Each Mirazid capsule contains 300mg of unstandardized myrrh extract. Several Egyptian studies have shown it to be effective in the treatment of schistosomiasis, a parasitic illness affecting millions of people around the globe. However, other studies have failed to show the same promising results. More investigation into dosage, frequencies, myrrh species and potencies may allow us to fine tune a more consistent positive parasitical cure rate especially since the parasite is developing a resistance toward the standard pharmaceuticals of choice.

Parts used: Resin

Global summary:
Used to treat: poor circulation, dysmenorrhea (difficult menstruation), postpartum pains secondary to stagnant blood, uterine tumors, infections of the mouth, gums, teeth, throat, stomach, syphilis, low energy, dyspepsia (digestive difficulties), diarrhea, obesity, hyperlipidemia (high cholesterol), atherosclerosis, bronchitis, asthma, coughing (difficulty bringing up mucus), diabetes, wounds, pain, dry and aging skin, parasites, vaginal inflammation, inflamed hemorrhoids, certain cancers (prostate), arthritis, osteoarthritis and rheumatism.
Used as a(n): 'spiritual tonic', tonic (stimulant), astringent, beautifying agent, emmanogogue (stimulating menstruation), stimulant of mucus membranes, stimulant of gastric juices,

expectorant, antioxidant, anti-tumor, anti-inflammatory, antiviral, antibacterial, antifungal, anti-parasitical, analgesic, antiseptic, and rejuvenating agent.

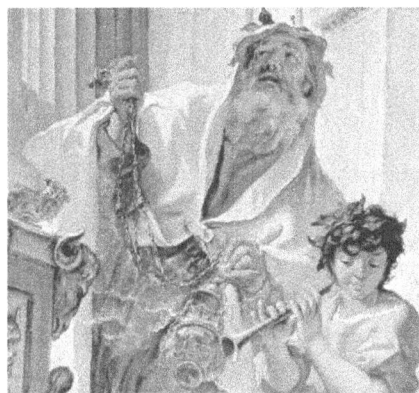

Ricci, Sebastiano, ca. 1700-1704 Italy

Summary medicinal uses and properties supported by scientific studies:
Antimicrobial, human heterophyiasis (intestinal fluke), schistosoma mansoni (flatworm), dicrocoeliasis dendriticum (small liver fluke), antiseptic, anesthetic, antitumor, anti-inflammatory, arthritis, apoptosis (destruction of various cancer cells), human fascioliasis (liver fluke – trematode Fasciola hepatica).

Egypt – Alexandria:
This study confirms the time-proven practice of using myrrh as an antimicrobial agent for a host of different diseases.[2]

Egypt – Cairo:
Another intestinal parasite, human heterophyiasis, has been destroyed with a 98% success rate using Mirazid (Commiphora molmol). Two capsules were given for a period of nine days before breakfast on an empty stomach.[3]

Egypt – Cairo:
According to this study, it would appear that myrrh could also be effec-

tive against another common parasite, schistosoma mansoni. Mice infected with this flatworm were given extract of myrrh (Mirazid), which in turn produced a significant reduction in worm and worm eggs.[4]

Egypt - Cairo:
In yet another study Mirazid was tested against the parasite, trematode Fasciola hepatica, a liver fluke causing human fascioliasis, which is spread to herbivores and humans alike through consuming infested aquatic plants or water. The infestations can produce abdominal pain (especially on the right upper abdomen - liver), generalized weakness, fever and nausea. More than 1,000 individuals were tested for the parasite. Those who tested positive were given two capsules with mirazil before breakfast for six days. The authors of the study reported: "The parasitological cure rate, two and three months after treatment, was 88.2% and 94.1% with an overt clinical cure without any side-effects."[5]

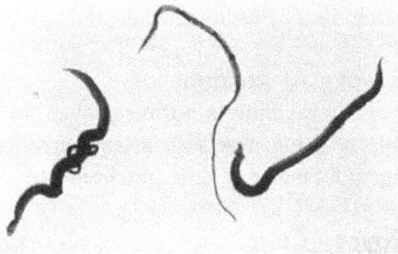

Schistosoma Mansonii. Courtesy: U.S. Center for Disease Control (CDC)

Egypt - El Mansurah:
Praziquantel has been the pharmaceutical drug of choice in the treatment of schistosomiasis. However, the parasite has become increasingly tolerant of the drug, which is also relatively expensive

(eight tablets cost about $50). In addition, it can produce serious side effects such as nausea, vomiting, dizziness, generalized weakness, headaches, fevers, muscle pains, cardiac arrhythmias and seizures. In this study, myrrh was given to 204 infected patients at a dose of 10mg/kg for a period of 3 days, which induced a cure rate of over 90% with mild and temporary side effects in some cases.[6] One hundred (500 – 600mg) capsules of myrrh costs about $4 – 6 in the U.S. and is most likely less expensive in countries closer to myrrh sources.

German Commission E:
Approved for the topical treatment of mucus membrane inflammation such as in sore throats.

Saudi Arabia - Jeddah:
Dicrocoeliasis dendriticum, or small liver fluke, is a parasite that most commonly affects sheep but to a lesser degree also humans. This study discovered that myrrh extract (600mg) from Commiphora molmol (syn. with C. myrrha) given before breakfast on an empty stomach for a period of six days produced a 100% success rate.[7] A stool analysis conducted as a follow up for all patients showed no signs of the fluke.

United States - Bethesda:
Based on traditional practice and evidence-based discoveries this researcher reported that myrrh's significant antiseptic, anesthetic, and antitumor properties are most likely attributed to a specific alkene called furanosesquiterpene, present in essential oil of myrrh.[8]

United States - Cincinnati:
This study discovered some of the potential physiological reasons why myrrh

has been used for thousands of years in the treatment of arthritis. Among the compounds tested, myrrh was able to modulate inflammatory responses.[9]

United States – Houston:
Scientists discovered that naturally occurring steroids (guggulsterone) from a closely related species called Commiphora mukul was able to produce apoptosis (destruction of cancer cells); "…including leukemia, head and neck carcinoma, multiple myeloma, lung carcinoma, melanoma, breast carcinoma, and ovarian carcinoma. Guggulsterone also inhibited the proliferation of drug-resistant cancer cells (e.g., gleevac-resistant leukemia, dexamethasone-resistant multiple myeloma, and doxorubicin-resistant breast cancer cells)."[10]

PREPARATIONS:
Myrrh comes in various grades of resin granules, powders, in capsule form, essential oil, and as a tincture.

Decoction: To enhance circulation, fight off microbes and to ease pain, use 3 - 6gm of myrrh, add two cups of cold water, bring to a boil, let it cool until warm, and drink up to two cups daily for up to 5 days.

Topical pain: Brake myrrh into a fine powder mix with coconut oil and apply to area of pain.

Parasites: Use on empty stomach.

Unwanted Effects:
Allergic reactions or contact dermatitis have been recorded upon contact with the skin in people with high sensitivity. Rapid heartbeats and kidney pains have been noted in some cases. Be careful if you are suffering from kidney disease and heart conditions prone to tachycardia (rapid heartbeats).

WARNING:
Do not use when pregnant; myrrh is used to bring about menstruation.

Sudan – Khartoum:
Department of Veterinary Medicine scientists tested various dosages of myrrh on goats. They discovered that a usage of 250mg/kg daily was nontoxic to the goats, while dosages of more than 1gm/kg daily and 5 gm/kg daily caused "grinding of teeth, salivation, soft feces, inappetence (lack of appetite), jaundice, dyspnea (difficulty breathing), ataxia (difficulty walking) and recumbency. Death occurred between 5 and 16 days. Organ examination found toxicity at kidneys and liver."[11]

Possible interaction with drugs:
Myrrh may increase the effectiveness of sugar metabolism and should thereby be used very carefully when using insulin or other diabetic controlling drugs. Consult with your healthcare provider prescribing the diabetic medication.

India –Mumbai:
Scientists determined in this study that a common Ayurvedic product, guggul lipid used to lower cholesterol, reduces the bioavailability of propranolol and diltiazem (valium). Patients receiving such beta-blockers and hypnotics should consider consulting with their respective healthcare professional.[12]

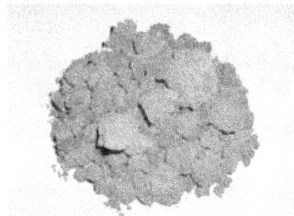

Courtesy: 'Gaius Cornelius'

1 Herodotus. Book II.73.

2 El Ashry ES, Rashed N, Salama OM, Saleh A. *Components, therapeutic value and uses of myrrh.* Chemistry Department, Faculty of Science, Alexandria University, Alexandria, Egypt. eelashry60@hotmail.com Pharmazie. 2003 Mar;58(3):163-8.

3 Massoud AM, El-Shazly AM, Morsy TA. *Mirazid (Commiphora molmol) in treatment of human heterophyiasis.* Department of Tropical Medicine, Faculty of Medicine, AI-Azhar University, Cairo, Egypt. J Egypt Soc Parasitol. 2007 Aug;37(2):395-410.

4 Hamed MA, Hetta MH. *Efficacy of Citrus reticulata and Mirazid in treatment of Schistosoma mansoni.* Department of Medicinal Chemistry, National Research Centre, Dokki, Cairo, Egypt. manal_hamed@yahoo.com Mem Inst Oswaldo Cruz. 2005 Nov;100(7):771-8.

5 Abo-Madyan AA, Morsy TA, *Motawea SM, Morsy AT. Clinical trial of Mirazid in treatment of human fascioliasis*, Ezbet El-Bakly (Tamyia Center) Al-Fayoum Governorate. Department of Tropical Medicine, Faculty of Medicine, Cairo University, Cairo, Egypt. J Egypt Soc Parasitol. 2004 Dec;34(3):807-18.

6 Sheir Z, Nasr AA, Massoud A, Salama O, Badra GA, El-Shennawy H, Hassan N, Hammad SM. *A safe, effective, herbal antischistosomal therapy derived from myrrh.* Department of Internal Medicine, Faculty of Medicine, Students' University Hospital, Mansoura University, Egypt. Am J Trop Med Hyg. 2001 Dec;65(6):700-4.

7 Al-Mathal EM, Fouad MA. *Myrrh (Commiphora molmol) in treatment of human and sheep dicrocoeliasis dendriticum in Saudi Arabia.* Department of Zoology, College of Science for Girls, Dammam, King Abdel-Aziz University, P.O. Box 80205, Jeddah 21589, Saudi Arabia. mathalem@hotmail.com J Egypt Soc Parasitol. 2004 Aug;34(2):713-20.

8 Nomicos EY. *Myrrh: medical marvel or myth of the magi?* National Institute of Allergy and Infectious Diseases, National Institute of Health, Bethesda, Maryland. Holist Nurs Pract. 2007 Nov-Dec;21(6):308-23.

9 Khanna D, Sethi G, Ahn KS, Pandey MK, Kunnumakkara AB, Sung B, Aggarwal A, Aggarwal BB. *Natural products as a gold mine for arthritis treatment.* Division of Immunology, Department of Medicine, University of Cincinnati, Cincinnati, OH, USA. Curr Opin Pharmacol. 2007 Jun;7(3):344-51.

10 Shishodia S, Sethi G, Ahn KS, Aggarwal BB. *Guggulsterone inhibits tumor cell proliferation, induces S-phase arrest, and promotes apoptosis through activation of c-Jun N-terminal kinase, suppression of Akt pathway, and downregulation of antiapoptotic gene products.* Cytokine Research Laboratory, Department of Experimental Therapeutics, Unit 143, The University of Texas M. D. Anderson Cancer Center, 1515 Holcombe Boulevard, Houston, TX 77030, United States. Biochem Pharmacol. 2007 Jun 30;74(1):118-30.

11 Omer SA, Adam SE. *Toxicity of Commiphora myrrha to goats.* Department of Veterinary Medicine, Pharmacology and Toxicology, University of Khartoum, Sudan. Vet Hum Toxicol. 1999 Oct;41(5):299-301.

12 Dalvi SS, Nayak VK, Pohujani SM, Desai NK, Kshirsagar NA, Gupta KC. *Effect of gugulipid on bioavailability of diltiazem and propranolol.* Dept of Pharmacology, Seth GS Medical College, Parel, Bombay. J Assoc Physicians India. 1994 Jun;42(6):454-5.

Amharic: Kerbe
Dutch: Mirre
French: Myrrhe
German: Myrrhe
Hebrew: Mor
Hindi: Bol
Homeopathic: Myrrh (Myrrh)
Italian: Mirra
Latin: Commiphora myrrha
Russian: Mnppa
Somali: Molmol
Spanish: Mirra
Tigrinya: Kerbe

Growth: Myrrh is a small tree or shrub that grows up to 4 meters (12 feet) in height.

Native to: East Africa, Namibia and the Southern Arabian Peninsula.

How to grow myrrh: The myrrh tree is a very tough plant and appears to love a solitary life the kind that can be found in the rocky desert landscapes of Namibia, Somalia, Oman or Ethiopia. The plant can handle the fierce sun and the little and only occasional water on top of rocky, sandy soil which makes it pretty much impossible to have any companions nearby. Myrrh trees that produce potent resign cannot be farmed but need to grow wild. In actuality very little is known and reported about how to grow the myrrh tree. Even though it is a valuable crop, there are no myrrh plantations, which speaks to the difficulty of man-made propagation.

If you are able to obtain some seeds plant a dozen or so about an inch apart in a spiral fashion about half an inch deep into a one-gallon clay pot. If you have more than one seed sprouting support the strongest one or separate them into individual pots. Try to re-create the plants environment. Find a solitary spot that provides bright light and plenty of warmth. If the roots reach the base transplant the plant into a larger container. Once the tree is established you may end up changing pots every year or so. Water the plant lightly and let the soil dry out completely in between. The plant will want to hibernate during the winter and may appear withered. Do not water during this time. Let it rest and begin to support the plant with the arrival of spring.

Time to seed: Late spring and well into the summer time. Collect seeds when you see the flowers wilting away. Keep them dry and dark until you are ready to seed.

Sun: Full, bright sun and heat.

Zone: 11-12. Low temperatures in Khartoum, Sudan average about 15°C.

Soil: Grows best in native, gravel like, desert soil. If you are growing the plant in pots, use clay, sand and a bit of gravel and mix well.

Harvest: While some of the resign oozes forth spontaneously, most of the myrrh resign is forced from the tree by tapping or incisions, about 5 cm in length, into the bark of a mature tree. The resign oozes out in tears and hardens a bit and is collected by the men during the beginning of hottest time of the year, which makes it a very difficult undertaking since they are collected by hand and the trees stand far apart. The cuts are repeated in the same spot on the bark for the next round of harvest. Collector transport the myrrh to caves in the mountains where they stay during the harvest until it is finished. The myrrh is than carefully moved by camel or donkey down from the mountains at night to the villages where it is dried in the shade for weeks and than carefully cleaned and sorted by the women. When this process is completed the myrrh is ready for sale.

Environmental concerns: Currently the self-regeneration of the myrrh trees is progressing very slowly. Scientists and collectors alike hypothesize that continued and intense tapping throughout the year may have reduced the trees ability to regenerate. To remedy the situation attempts are being made to implement a harvest limit and by providing alternating harvest breaks to enhance myrrh tree self-propagation.

Storage: Dried myrrh resign keeps for a long time when kept protected from moisture and the elements.

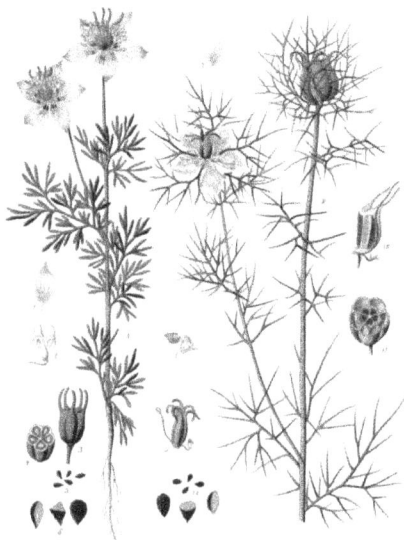

Köhler's Medicinal Plants 1887

Nigella

Breathe - You
are Alive

Black seed of nigella, which has sustained a 'spiritual' aura throughout the ages, can be found in a variety of cultures. An Arabian legend transmitted in Al-Hadith, an oral history of the words and deeds of the Islamic prophet Mohammad, tells of an herb that is: 'the medicine for every disease except death.' In Arabic, Habba Al-baraca means 'blessed seed'.

Nigella seeds are as black as a moonless night. In Sanskrit, nigella is Krishna jeeraka. Krishna, which is sanskrit for black, is the Hindi deity whose skin-color was dark enough to take on a blue-hue.

In the 11th century, Ibn Sina, known in the west by his Latin name Avicenna, wrote one of the most famous medicinal volumes, the Canon of Medicine, in which he prescribes nigella as a general stimulant and tonic for body and spirit.

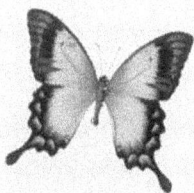

Breathe easy and breathe deep. Let life enter, let restrictions go. 'The world is a scary place' can go as easily as fear, anger and lingering pain. I take my power back from all that is restricting, and protect myself through forgiveness, gratitude, love for myself, remembering my worth and a lingering hope and diligent focus on the possibility of peace of mind.

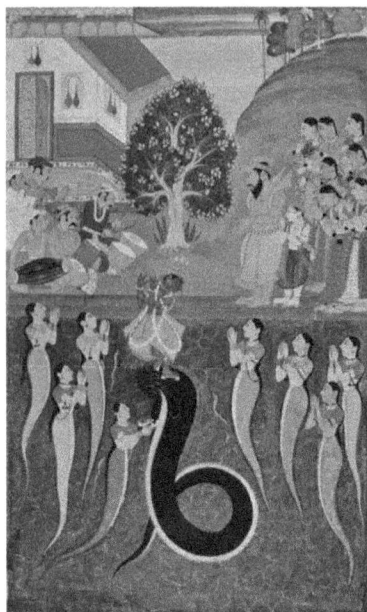

The blue Hindu god Krishna. Bhâgavata-Purâna-Manuskript. India 1640

Parts used: seeds and oils from seeds

Global summary:
Used to treat: allergies, asthma, bronchitis, colds, heart disease, inflammatory diseases, poor milk production in nursing mothers, digestive difficulties, skin problems, low immunity, poor digestion, parasites, diabetes, colon cancer. **Used as a(n):** antithelminic (destructive to parasites), carminative (reducing gas), digestive aid, diaphoretic, diuretic, emmenagogue (helps to assist menstruation), galactogogue (enhances mild production in lactating mothers), female breast size enhancer, antihypotensive, antibacterial, antifungal, analgesic, anti-inflammatory, bronchodilatory, immuno-potentiator, cardiac tonic.

Summary of medicinal uses and properties supported by scientific studies 2004 - 2007:
Possible prophylactic effect in asthma patients, bronchodilator, antihistaminic, relaxant, anticholinergic, anti-inflammatory, antiarthritic, antitumor, antidiabetic, may prevent kidney stones, antihypertensive, antibacterial, antifungal, analgesic, cardiac tonic, may destroy prostate cancer cells, may prevent prostate cancer, may prevent and treat colon cancer, protects against ionizing radiation, possible treatment and prevention of Schistosomiasis, and a possible anticonvulsant (seizure).

Egypt - Dokki:
Schistosomiasis (snail fever) is a parasitical disease caused by a flatworm carried by certain snails living in dammed waters or natural ponds. This common tropical illness affects millions of people worldwide. Egyptian scientists examined the possible role of black seeds

Let us examine black seed's reputation as a universal remedy for the body, mind and spirit. As of September 2007, the National Library of Medicine lists 176 published nigella studies in numerous international scientific journals.

Nigella, an annual, is easily propagated from seed. It grows well in North African countries but is cultivated as far southeast as Ethiopia where it is used to flavor local drinks. Black seed is used in many of northern India's vegetable recipes and as an ingredient for breads, such as naan in Peshawar, Pakistan, or Jewish rye bread in New York. The blessed seed, known for its almost omnipresent flavor in Arab bakery goods, can be ground and eaten mixed with honey.

There exists a common confusion about the name of this plant. To avoid using the wrong species, try to find a source that is certain about the Latin name nigella sativa.

in the treatment of Schistosomiasis and found that it possessed a strong ability to destroy the parasite in all stages of its life cycle. In addition, it created a hostile environment in the body for the parasitical egg implantation.[1] The study found a reduced production rate of oxidative enzymes. Is it this function that allows the body's own defense against parasites - cellular hydrogen peroxide - to destroy the worm?

Iran - Mashhad:
Doctors evaluated the extracts from boiled nigella seeds on asthmatic adults and determined that those patients using the extract reported a reduction in all asthma symptoms, including improved pulmonary function tests. Furthermore, patients experienced a reduced need for inhalers.[2]

In this rodent-model study from Mashad, scientists determined that alcoholic extracts of nigella sativa reduced calcium oxalate deposits (a main cause for kidney stone formation).[3] While more research is needed to determine if similar reduction occurs in humans it is a possible promising prophylactic especially in people familiar with the extreme pain of passing a kidney stone.

Another rodent study from Mashad determined that black seed had the ability to suppress epileptic seizures, in both reoccurence and severity, thus considering the possible anti-convulsant properties of the plant.[4]

Saudi Arabia - Dammam:
Two kinds of cardiac hypertrophy exist. One is pathological and produces a variety of heart problems; and the other is physiological, usually brought on by regular exercise, enhancing overall heart functions. King Faisal University

scientists discovered that rats, when fed 800mg/kg black seed over a period of two months, developed physiological cardiac hypertrophy. This, to date, is the first such study examining the potential of nigella for overall heart function and health.[5]

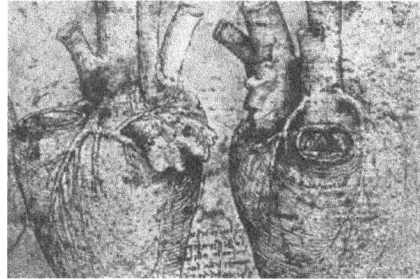

The heart. Leonardo daVinci, ca. 1510

Turkey - Zonguldak:
Human parathyroid hormone, a treatment for osteoporosis (an especially serious problem in patients with insulin dependent diabetes), has been found to significantly enhance its therapeutic abilities when combined with nigella extract.[6]

Turkey - Yüzüncü Yıl University:
Another study from Turkey demonstrated that the volatile oil of nigella can suppress artificially induced arthritis in rats, adding a bit more understanding as to the time-proven use of nigella in the treatment of arthritis and other similar chronic inflammatory conditions.[7]

Turkey - Afyon:
Ionizing radiation is used to treat many human cancer patients. However, the radiation does not discriminate between cancer cells and healthy cells, and, as a result, massive tissue damage across the board occurs. This study from Turkey, using a rodent model, found that the radiation damage to the healthy tissue

might be minimized by nigella sativa oil ingestion (1ml/kg body weight) and injections of glutathione. The study reports: "These results clearly show that NS and GSH treatment significantly antagonize the effects of radiation. Therefore, NS and GSH may be a beneficial agent in protection against ionizing radiation-related tissue injury."[8]

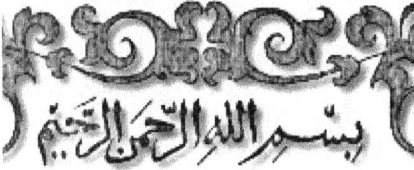

From a 1593 copy of Ibn Sina's Canon of Medicine. Courtesy: Beirut University

Morocco – Béni-Mellal:
Injecting nigella essential oil into the tumor sites significantly reduced solid tumor development, inhibited metastasis, and improved the overall survival of the test mice.[9]

United States – Detroit:
Scientists at the Henry Ford Hospital noted that a body of international reports, mostly from the Middle East and Asia, found nigella to have an antineoplastic (abnormal growth of cells of benign or cancerous tumors) effect in both the laboratory and real patients. They isolated a component of nigella called thymoquinone and tested it in a rodent model. They discovered that the nigella based compound produced apoptosis – the destruction of cancer cells without notable side effects. They also concluded that thymoquinone may also help prevent prostate cancer.[10]

United States – Jackson:
In a University of Mississippi Medical Center Jackson study, Mississippi scientists were following the reported time-proven threads from the Middle East. They examined the possible therapeutic effects of catechin, found in green tea, and thymoquinone, a major compound from black seed (nigella sativa), on specific colon cancer cells. They compared both natural products with the effectiveness of the current chemotherapeutic drug of choice - 5-fluorouracil - against colon cancer cell lines. Scientists determined that both the green tea – catechin - and the thymoquinone from nigella sativa "have demonstrated incredible chemotherapeutic responses,[11] thus suggesting that both may have similar chemotherapeutic effects as their pharmacological counterpart 5-fluorouracil, which has known serious side effects including cardiac toxicity."

PREPARATIONS:
Black seeds can be eaten plain: use one teaspoon; for a sweeter taste, use a bit of honey, or they can be sprinkled onto bread or pastries

Prepare a tea by boiling the black seed in water, strain and allow it to cool down; drink a few cups a day.

Some prefer to use the ground seeds mixed with water or raw organic milk.

Preparations are available in gelatin capsules (500mg). Take 1-2 daily.

Unwanted Effects: N/A

WARNING:
Do not use during pregnancy.

Possible interaction with drugs:
Enhances the increased bone density effect of human parathyroid hormone.

1 Mohamed AM, Metwally NM, Mahmoud SS. *Sativa seeds against Schistosoma mansoni different stages.* Department of Medicinal Chemistry, National Research Centre, Dokki, Egypt. Azzanrc@hotmail.com Mem Inst Oswaldo Cruz. 2005 Apr;100(2):205-11.

2 Boskabady MH, Javan H, Sajady M, Rakhshandeh H. *The possible prophylactic effect of Nigella sativa seed extract in asthmatic patients.* Department of Physiology, Ghaem Medical Centre, Mashhad University of Medical Sciences, Mashhad 91735, Iran. Fundam Clin Pharmacol. 2007 Oct;21(5):559-66.

3 Hadjzadeh MA, Khoei A, Hadjzadeh Z, Parizady M. *Ethanolic extract of nigella sativa L seeds on ethylene glycol-induced kidney calculi in rats.* Department of Physiology, Ghaem Hospital, Mashhad University of Medical Sciences, Mashhad, Iran. Urol J. 2007 Spring;4(2):86-90.

4 Hosseinzadeh H, Parvardeh S, Nassiri-Asl M, Mansouri MT. *Intracerebroventricular administration of thymoquinone, the major constituent of Nigella sativa seeds, suppresses epileptic seizures in rats.* Department of Pharmacodynamics & Toxicology, Faculty of Pharmacy, Mashhad University of Medical Sciences, Mashhad, Iran. hosseinzadehh@yahoo.com Med Sci Monit. 2005 Apr;11(4):BR106-10.

5 El-Bahai MN, Al-Hariri MT, Yar T, Bamosa AO. *Cardiac inotropic and hypertrophic effects of Nigella sativa supplementation in rats.* Department of Physiology, College of Medicine, King Faisal University, PO Box 2114, Dammam, 31451, Saudi Arabia. Int J Cardiol. 2007 Oct 9.

6 Altan MF. *Effects of Nigella sativa and Human Parathyroid Hormone on Bone Mass and Strength in Diabetic Rats.* Department of Civil Engineering, Faculty of Engineering, Zonguldak Karaelmas University, Zonguldak, Turkey. Biol Trace Elem Res. 2007 Jun;116(3):321-8.

7 Tekeoglu I, Dogan A, Ediz L, Budancamanak M, Demirel A. *Effects of thymoquinone (volatile oil of black cumin) on rheumatoid arthritis in rat models.* Yuzuncu Yil University, Medical School, Department of Rehabilitation and Rheumatology, Turkey. Phytother Res. 2007 Sep;21(9):895-7.

8 Cemek M, Enginar H, Karaca T, Unak P. *In vivo radioprotective effects of Nigella sativa L oil and reduced glutathione against irradiation-induced oxidative injury and number of peripheral blood lymphocytes in rats.* Department of Chemistry, Biochemistry Division, Faculty of Science and Arts, Afyon Kocatepe University, Afyon, Turkey. mcemek@yahoo.com Photochem Photobiol. 2006 Nov-Dec;82(6):1691-6.

9 Ait Mbarek L, Ait Mouse H, Elabbadi N, Bensalah M, Gamouh A, Aboufatima R, Benharref A, Chait A, Kamal M, Dalal A, Zyad A. *Anti-tumor properties of blackseed (Nigella sativa L.) extracts.* Laboratory of Immunology, Biochemistry and Molecular Biology, Faculty of Sciences and Technologies, Cadi-Ayyad University, Béni-Mellal, Morocco. Braz J Med Biol Res. 2007 Jun;40(6):839-47.

10 Kaseb AO, Chinnakannu K, Chen D, Sivanandam A, Tejwani S, Menon M, Dou QP, Reddy GP. *Androgen receptor and E2F-1 targeted thymoquinone therapy for hormone-refractory prostate cancer.* Department of Hematology/Oncology, Henry Ford Hospital, MI 458202, USA. Cancer Res. 2007 Aug 15;67(16):7782-8.

11 Norwood AA, Tucci M, Benghuzzi H. *A comparison of 5-fluorouracil and natural chemotherapeutic agents, EGCG and thymoquinone, delivered by sustained drug delivery on colon cancer cells.* University of Mississippi Medical Center, 2500 North State Street, Jackson, Mississippi 39216, USA. Biomed Sci Instrum. 2007;43:272-7

Amharic: Tikur Azmud
Dutch: Nigelle
French: Nigelle, cumin noir
German: Schwarzkümmel
Hebrew: Ketzah
Hindi: Kalounji
Homeopathic: Nigella sativa (Nig-s.)
Italian: Grano nero
Korean: Nigella
Latin: Nigella sativa
Russian: Nigella
Sanskrit: Krishna jeeraka
Spanish: Neguilla

Growth: Nigella is a hardy, annual, flowering, hermaphrodite that can grow up about 1 foot high and wide.

Native to: Arabia, East Africa, Mediterranean and Western Asia.

How to grow nigella: Black seed is easy to grow from seed. Buy some organic seed and place them directly into soil after the last frost has passed. Place the seeds a ¼ inch deep and cover them lightly with soil. Moisten the seedbed slightly but do not over water. Once the plant is established it is quite drought tolerant and can get by with little water. Thinning of rows maybe necessary. Plants can also be transplanted. Remember the plant is self-seeding, especially if you have no frost during winter.

Time to seed: In Spring

Sun: Full sun and warm location preferred, the plant does not like shade.

Zone: 7 – 10

Soil: Well-drained clay based, sandy soil but will tolerate most any good garden soil. The application of some nitrogen may enhance the therapeutic properties of the plant.

Harvest: Seeds ripen in fall. Allow the fruits to mature and dry on the plant. Immature fruits contain white seed kernel. Mature fruits are dry and when begin to crack open and offer up their content fully turned black seeds. Collect them and clean off the fruit capsule and wilted flower leafs.

Attracts friends: Bees, lacewing, hummingbirds and butterflies.

Environmental benefits: Dried black seeds are placed loosely in small cotton sacks, which are than placed in between woolen clothing to prevent insects from making a meal of it.

Storage: Store them in a dry and dark container for you usage or reseeding next spring.

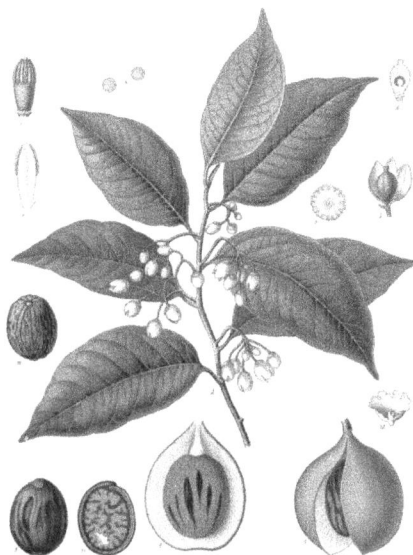

Köhler's Medicinal Plants 1887

Nutmeg

Shrouded in the mists of time lies a mystery. Mystery gives birth to wonder; wonder transcends fear. Let the adventure begin.

According to historical records, the nutmeg tree, myristica fragrans, originated on few relatively small Indonesian islands. (Myristicus is Greek for "smelling like Myrr.") While Indian and Arabian traders brought nutmeg to North Africa and eventually Europe, they were still able to keep the islands' origin a secret for many centuries. Nevertheless, Genoa and Ven- ice built their riches on trade with this seed born from an almost mythical land in an exotic paradise. Its mystique matched its expense, which was comparable to gold at the time. Thus, by the 17th century, the Dutch East India Company (V.O.C.) had muscled a monopo- ly, which helped propel it into one of the largest corporate entities of that time. The beautiful city

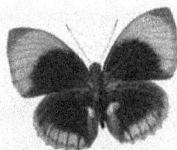

There is more to life than meets the eye; there are colors beyond black; and there are colors beyond white that can touch, protect you, nurture you, ease your pain, lift you and support you. I can help you to stay awake in the knowledge that you are more than capable of receiving what nurtures you and reject what retards your growth, your beauty and your fun.

of Amsterdam also owes much of its lasting beauty to a little mysterious seed valued by Roman emperors, European royalties and Marco Polo alike. In turn, nutmeg owes its value to part of a century-long secret dearly kept by Indian and Arabian traders.

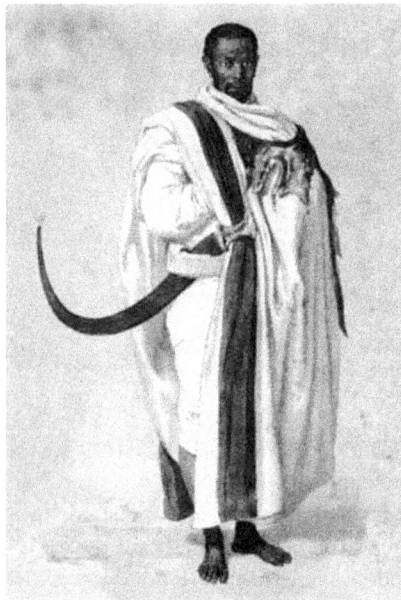

T. Lefebvre. Voyage en Abyssinie. 1845

Some of this popularity was perhaps also based on her hallucinogenic properties, which some found enjoyable but others most found difficult. (Medium to high dose experiences are very unpredictable.) Those who could afford the alluring seed burned it during important celebrations in homes and streets. What is it that makes nutmeg at higher doses so unpredictable? What is it that made nutmeg a co-creator to the beauty and power of the trade cities of long ago?

Another reason for nutmeg's European popularity was its professed ability to cure the plague, which had already deci-mated half of Europe's population. History hints that none knew the plagues' origins. Various theories continue to be proposed today. If, indeed, a bacteria was involved, some of nutmeg's anti-bacterial properties might have had a positive impact, which indeed would explain the huge amount of interest and money spent at the time on this spice.

The tree produces a shiny black seed kernel, which is surrounded by a bright red and web like mace layer - both of which have potent bioactive properties. Once the mace and seed are separated and dried the seed turns into a sand color with a hard appearance commonly sold in today's stores.

Nutmeg exemplifies a natural food spice that exhibits both powerfully mind-altering and medicinal properties - depending on the dosage used. The spice carries an age-old reputation of producing a menstrual period and inducing abortions, and easing indigestion and diarrhea. This has led, in part, to reported overdoses where people enter altered mental and emotional states similar to those described with alcoholic or psychedelic experiences. Users may undergo a variety of effects, including: a total lack of control from hysteria to malaise, nausea, vomiting, dizziness, amnesia, near death experiences, enhanced endurance, heightened sensual experiences, extraordinary visions, exhilaration, clairvoyance or a sense of being in two places at once.

In homeopathy, extremely diluted solutions of nutmeg are used to treat many of the very symptoms the tree's seed causes in its crude and over-dosed state. It is considered a key remedy in cases where one or more signs and symptoms correspond and match a patient's overall case study. Keynote symptoms for the possible selection of nux moschata as a remedy include in part: confusion, foolishness, extreme mood changes, sense of being two people, loss of memory, things seeming unreal, dry mucus membranes (eyes, mouth, constipation but without being thirsty) and fighting to stay awake.

Since the 15th century, the Portuguese managed to find the Indonesian islands, and within a short period of time the nutmeg plants had been stolen and shipped to other tropical countries under their control. Today, nutmeg lists as a major crop in many tropical countries. Grenada's economy and unique healing tradition depends much on nutmeg, so much so that a likeness of the seed has been incorporated into the country's flag.

Parts used: The dried seed kernels and mace layer surrounding the seed.

Global summary:
Used to treat: Pain, sprains and strains, diarrhea, lack of appetite, skin problems such as puss-filled boils or eczema, heart disease, digestive difficulties, gas, indigestion, poor appetite, nausea, oxidative stress, asthma, inflammation, fever, rheumatism, arthritis, high blood pressure, oral infection, insomnia, diabetes, lymphatic congestion, kidney problems, depression, loss of memory, heart burn, stroke, missing menstruation, mild depression

Used as a(n): hallucinogenic, clairvoyant, sedative, analgesic, smooth muscle relaxant, appetite stimulant, digestive, anti-inflammatory, antibacterial, cardiac tonic, emaciation, antioxidant and antispasmodic.

Summary medicinal uses and properties supported by scientific studies:
Acts as a male aphrodisiac, possible anti-depressant and mood enhancer, possible memory enhancer, possible memory loss protector; is radio-protective, anti-bacterial, cholesterol lowering, a heartburn inhibitor, anti-thrombotic (reduces blood clotting); may enhance insulin metabolism, prevent tooth decay (anti caries); has psychoactive components (various alkaloids); and, is possibly helpful in type 2 diabetes associated with obesity.

India – Aligarh:
Unani traditions boast nutmeg's longstanding reputation as a male aphrodisiac. Now an Aligarh Muslim University study may provide further clues into why nutmeg aides in the treatment of male sexual dysfunctions. The researchers noted that when rats were given a 50% alcoholic extract of nutmeg as well as clove (500mg/kg), male rats experienced an increased sexual appetite without any noticeable side effects.[1]

India – Hisar:
An extract of nutmeg seeds (10mg/kg) has been found - in a mouse model - to have anti-depressant properties similar to those of pharmacological anti-depressants like imipramine (15 mg/kg) and fluoxetine (20 mg/kg). The researchers from Guru Jambheshwar University in Hisar state: "The antidepressant-like effect of the extract seems to be mediated by interaction with the adrenergic, dopaminergic, and serotonergic systems."[2]

India – Hisar:
Various constituents of nutmeg were extracted from the dried powder of the seed and applied against a variety of gram-positive and gram-negative

bacteria. Researchers from the Department of Pharmaceutical Sciences, Guru Jambheshwar University, in Hisar, determined that all extracted constituents exhibited good anti-bacterial activities, which could be used to replace synthetic preservatives.[3]

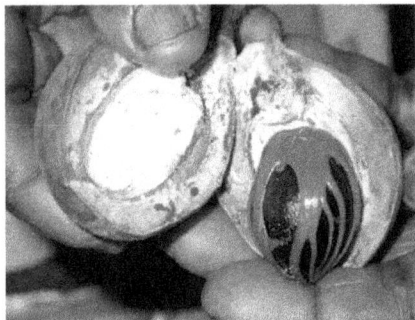

Nutmeg shell, seed kernel and mace. Grenada.

India - Hisar:

This particular study presents more of nutmeg's potentially mind-affecting properties. A mouse model revealed that an extract from the plant's seed given at 5mg/kg over a period of 3 days could enhance memory function in the rodents. In addition, the extract protected the mice from the impairment, which the scientists had tried to produce in them with doses of scopolamine and diazepam.[4]

India - Jaipur:

University of Rajasthan scientists evaluated a completely different therapeutic property of nutmeg, which may protect against the damaging effects of gamma radiation.[5] Gamma radiation resembles x-ray emissions - the major difference being its source. Both are ionizing radiations that penetrate the skin, possibly producing changes in the DNA of each cell. These permutations can result in a variety of cancers and congenital conditions, which may be passed on to

following generations.

India - Jaipur:

In this study, scientists fed rabbits an alcoholic extract of nutmeg at 500mg/kg for a period of 60 days. Rabbits significantly experienced reduced cholesterol in the heart and liver and improved ability in reducing blood clots.[6]

Korea - Yusong-gu:

Korean scientists explored the use of an isolated nutmeg extract in the treatment of Type 2 Diabetes and obesity. Scientists discovered that the extract inhibited a certain protein expression, thereby enhancing insulin signals inside the cells.[7]

Korea - Seoul:

In this study, Korean scientists isolated a nutmeg compound called macelignan, which has strong anti-bacterial properties especially when tested against caries (tooth decay). The compound also produced the bacteria Streptococcus mutans.[8]

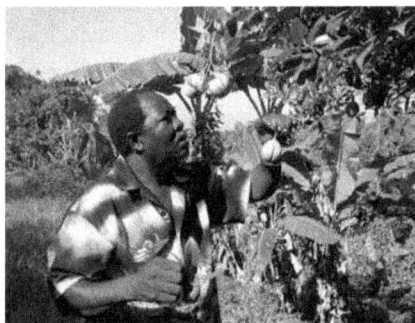

Keith Whint and the Nutmeg tree. Grenada.

Keith Whint, one of Grenada's own, believes the use of oral nutmeg in any form may help in cases of strokes. He says it may buy more time and reduce the flow of internal blood loss while the victim is quickly taken to the nearest hospital.

Nigeria - Ibadan:

A Nigerian study discovered that nutmeg has antithrombotic properties. Perhaps Keith Whint's story about nutmeg in cases of strokes is based on some of these recent discoveries.

Pakistan - Saidu Sharif

In a study from Pakistan, scientists found that Verapamil, a calcium channel blocker used to slow down prolonged rapid heartbeats as well as high blood pressure, also functions similarly to cimetidine in reducing gastric juices.[9] These same scientists found nutmeg to perform similarly.

A separate study from this same Saidu Department of Pharmacology determined that nutmeg also reduced gastric juices, but without the side effects.[10]

PREPARATIONS:

It is best to only buy the whole seeds and grind them for culinary purposes as needed. One reason includes freshness and potency. The other contends that unscrupulous producers have used moldy and rotten seeds to prepare the powdered spice, which still may contain mold and the possible toxins they produce.

Nutmeg oil is commonly used topically in Grenada in the treatment of arthritis, rheumatism, and sprains and strains.

Capsules are available from a variety of suppliers. Try to find a reputable source to assure only good quality seeds have been used. Use 500mg to 1gm two to three times a day for indigestion, dyspepsia and flatulence.

Unwanted Effects:

The effects of moderate to high doses (5-20gm) of dried nutmeg can vary extremely and are quite unpredictable. Nausea, vomiting, panic attacks, rapid heartbeats, diarrhea, 'cotton-mouth', dry mucus membranes, constipation, dry eyes, and drowsiness are often reported when used at dosages approaching the psychedelic/sedative effects. The onset of symptoms may not occur until several hours after ingestion and may last up to three to seven days with decreasing intensity after about 24 hours of primary and possible significant hallucinogenic effects.

WARNING:

Psychotropic experiences at high doses have been reported. Nutmeg overdoses cannot be detected in urine.[11] It is thought that the main suspected psychotropic ingredients (elemicin, myristicin and safrole) contribute to the formation of an amphetamine-like derivative as part of the body's metabolic process.

Poison control centers in Texas received 17 calls involving nutmeg ingestion between 1998 and 2004. Reports stipulate that the majority were intentional nutmeg abuse ingestions or that of intentional and unintentional use: "None of the ingestions resulted in more than moderate clinical effects or death."[12]

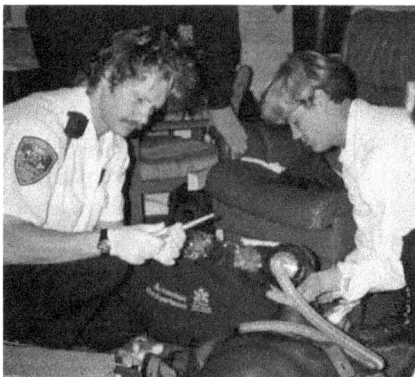

Author Injecting an Overdose Victim with an Antidote, San Francisco 1995

Do not drive when under the influence of nutmeg. Depending on dose, individual tolerance and metabolism, effects may last up to a week.

German Commission E:

As of 1986, nutmeg was considered an unapproved drug due to the risk versus benefit analysis. The Commission reports that high doses can cause abortions. It urges caution.

Sweden - Uppsala:

This study suggests that human intoxication has been reported at approximately 5gm of nutmeg seed, which corresponds to about 1-2 mg myristicin/kg body weight.[13] Myristicin is the principal aromatic constituent of nutmeg's volatile oil.

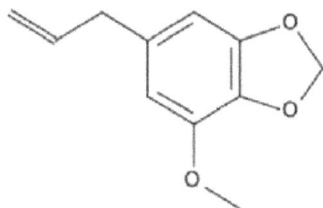

Myristicin

Possible interaction with drugs:

According to the German Commission E, nutmeg acts as a monoamine oxidase inhibitor (MAOI) blocking prostaglandin synthesis.[14] While currently no studies exist to determine nutmeg's interaction with pharmaceutical medications, it may be possible that nutmeg interferes with a group of anti-depressant drugs also containing MAOI. Monoamine oxidase is a naturally occurring enzyme in the human body. It is responsible for the break down of presently no longer needed neurotransmitters, such as serotonin or norepinepherine. MAOIs suppress this enzyme, which in turn extends the time interval of neurotransmitters such as serotine, norepinepherine and dopamine in the circulation. This allows for a prolonged effect of physiological and emotional impacts, such as mood elevation. It may be possible for MAOI's action to be fortified and enhanced by using MAOI drugs and nutmeg, thus allowing for decreased risk of side effects. Some common side effects: dizziness, dry mouth, sensation of drunkenness, constipation, hypotension and reduced sexual interest. Some serious side effects of MAOIs: severe anxiety, dizziness, rapid heartbeats, diaphoresis (sweating), panic attacks, seizures, fever, hallucinations, and shortness of breath.

Inhibition of prostaglandin production may lead to a wide variety of biological functions related to prostaglandin. Different tissue experiences caused varied affects from prostaglandin, making it a versatile substance in controlling pain, inflammation and glandular secretion. Prostaglandin, which has hormone-like effects, is involved in: smooth muscle contraction, lowered blood pressure, and stimulated uterine contractions and blood vessels in the intestines. This may explain the age-old belief in nutmeg being able to abort a pregnancy.

1 Tajuddin , Ahmad S, Latif A, Qasmi IA. *Aphrodisiac activity of 50% ethanolic extracts of Myristica fragrans Houtt. (nutmeg) and Syzygium aromaticum (L) Merr. & Perry. (clove) in male mice: a comparative study.* Department of Ilmul Advia (Unani Pharmacology), Faculty of Unani Medicine, Aligarh Muslim University, Aligarh-202002, India. BMC Complement Altern Med. 2003 Oct 20;3:6.

2 Dhingra D, Sharma A. *Antidepressant-like*

activity of n-hexane extract of nutmeg (Myristica fragrans) seeds in mice. Pharmacology Division, Department of Pharmaceutical Sciences, Guru Jambheshwar University, Hisar, Haryana, India. J Med Food. 2006 Spring;9(1):84-9.

3 Narasimhan B, Dhake AS. Antibacterial principles from Myristica fragrans seeds. Department of Pharmaceutical Sciences, Guru Jambheshwar University, Hisar, Haryana, India. J Med Food. 2006 Fall;9(3):395-9.

4 Parle M, Dhingra D, Kulkarni SK. Improvement of mouse memory by Myristica fragrans seeds. Pharmacology Division, Department of Pharmaceutical Sciences, Guru Jambheshwar University, Hisar-125001, Haryana, India. mparle@rediffmail.com J Med Food. 2004 Summer;7(2):157-61.

5 Sharma M, Kumar M. Radioprotection of Swiss albino mice by Myristica fragrans houtt. Cell and Molecular Biology Lab, Department of Zoology, University of Rajasthan, Jaipur, India. J Radiat Res (Tokyo). 2007 Mar;48(2):135-41.

6 Ram A, Lauria P, Gupta R, Sharma VN. Hypolipidaemic effect of Myristica fragrans fruit extract in rabbits. Department of Pharmacology, S.M.S. Medical College, Jaipur, India. J Ethnopharmacol. 1996 Dec;55(1):49-53.

7 Yang S, Na MK, Jang JP, Kim KA, Kim BY, Sung NJ, Oh WK, Ahn JS. Inhibition of protein tyrosine phosphatase 1B by lignans from Myristica fragrans. Korea Research Institute of Bioscience and Biotechnology (KRIBB), 52 Eoeun-dong, Yusong-gu, Daejeon 305-333, Korea. Phytother Res. 2006 Aug;20(8):680-2.

8 Chung JY, Choo JH, Lee MH, Hwang JK. Anticariogenic activity of macelignan isolated from Myristica fragrans (nutmeg) against Streptococcus mutans. Department of Biomaterials Science and Engineering, Yonsei University, Seoul, South Korea. Phytomedicine. 2006 Mar;13(4):261-6.

9 Jan M, Orakzai SA, Tariq S, Javid M, Ahmad S, Haroon M, Qamar M. Comparison of verapamil and cimetidine for their effects on volume and acidity of Carbachol induced gastric secretion in fasting rabbits. Department of Pharmacology, Saidu Medical College, Swat, Pakistan. J Ayub Med Coll Abbottabad. 2005 Jul-Sep;17(3):11-4.

10 Jan M, Faqir F, Hamida , Mughal MA. Comparison of effects of extract of Myristica fragrans and verapamil on the volume and acidity of carbachol induced gastric secretion in fasting rabbits. Department of Pharmacology SMC, Swat, Saidu Sharif, Pakistan. J Ayub Med Coll Abbottabad. 2005 Apr-Jun;17(2):69-71.

11 Beyer J, Ehlers D, Maurer HH. Abuse of nutmeg (Myristica fragrans Houtt.): studies on the metabolism and the toxicologic detection of its ingredients elemicin, myristicin, and safrole in rat and human urine using gas chromatography/mass spectrometry. Department of Experimental and Clinical Toxicology, Institute of Experimental and Clinical Pharmacology and Toxicology, University of Saarland, Homburg (Saar), Germany. Ther Drug Monit. 2006 Aug;28(4):568-75.

12 Forrester MB. Nutmeg intoxication in Texas, 1998-2004. Epidemiology and Disease Surveillance Unit, Texas Department of State Health Services, Austin 78756, USA. Hum Exp Toxicol. 2005 Nov;24(11):563-6.

13 Hallström H, Thuvander A. Toxicological evaluation of myristicin. Division of Toxicology, National Food Administration, Uppsala, Sweden. heha@msmail.slv.se Nat Toxins. 1997;5(5):186-92.

14 Mark Blumenthal, Werner R. Busse, Alicia Goldberg, Joerg Grenwald, Tara Hall, Chance W. Riggins, Robert S. Rister. The Complete German Commission E Monographs: Therapeutic Guide to Herbal Medicines. Bundesinstitut fur Arzneimittel und Medizinprodukte (Germany). 1st English edition published by Lippincott Williams & Wilkins; (August 15, 1998).

Amharic: Gabz
Dutch: Nootmuskaat
French: Muscade
German: Muskat
Hebrew: Muskat
Hindi: Taifal
Homeopathic:Nux moschata (Nux-m.)
Italian: Moscata
Korean: Notumek
Latin: Myristica fragrans
Russian: Muskatny
Sanskrit: Jatiphala
Spanish: Moscada
Tigrinya: Sigem

Growth: Nutmeg is an evergreen tropical tree that can reach a height of about 60 feet.

Native to: Molucca (spice) islands of Indonesia. Today Indonesia and the Caribbean island Grenada are the principle producers of nutmeg, but it is also grown to a significant degree in Sri Lanka, India and Malaysia.

How to grow nutmeg: This tree species require a male and a female tree to grow nutmeg seeds. Collect the ripe seeds, ideally from trees that have shown a high yield in seed production, just as they are falling down by themselves or when their green/yellow outer shell is beginning to split revealing the mace and seed. Remove the fleshy outer layer as well as the bright red mace layer from the seed. It is best to plant the seeds as soon as possible. Fresher seed tend to have a higher germination rate. Prepare a shallow seedbed with a good mix of organic soil, sand and some manure. Place the seeds into the soil and cover them but slightly. Keep the bed moist but not wet. Germination may take between 1-3 months. Separate the sprouted seedling into approximate 3-gallon containers and keep them until they have well established root systems, stem and foliage. This can take between 1 and 2 years. Nutmeg grows well in a mixed garden that contains banana, cocoa, palm trees, coconut and other diffused shade providing tropical trees.

Time to seed: As the trees are falling from the tree or the outer shell begins to split.

Sun: Diffused and continuous shade is especially important for young nutmeg trees.

Zone: 11 or higher.

Soil: Well drained nutrient rich organic, clay and sand containing soil. Add frequent manure to assure a healthy plant.

Harvest: The tree announces its own harvest. When the seed begin to fall. It may take up to 6 – 7 years for the tree to reach the maturity needed to produce nutmegs. The seeds are collected and dried, single layer in the sun. The outer layer is removed and the mace is separated and also dried in the sun. The black seed kernel is broken with a mallet when the inside seed is loose enough to make a sound when shaken. What is left is the nutmeg. It is sold as a nutmeg or ground and sold as a powder.

Attracts friends: Bees and other pollinating insects and animals.

Environmental benefits: Nutmeg trees do well in diverse and organic gardens that have shown, especially on Grenada, to support a whole family with year around sustainable food production for consumption and sale.

Storage: Nutmeg as nut or powder stored in a dry and dark environment can stay potent for a very long time.

ORIGANUM
VULGARE

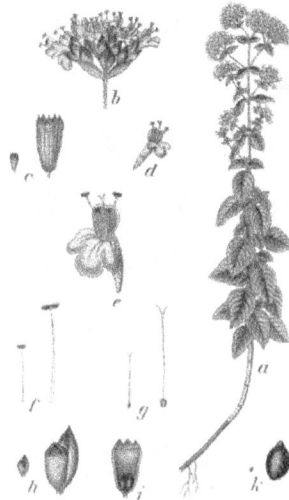

Oregano

Johann Georg Sturm & Painter Jacob Sturm, Germany 1796

There is light
and there is
shadow on
the mountain
of Aphrodite
from whence
I came.

It is said in Greece that Oregano was bestowed as a gift from the goddess of love herself – Aphrodite. The name may be derived from the Greek oros (mountain) and agapo (love). Some speculate that the biblical hyssop was a species of oregano. "Purge me with hyssop, and I shall be clean..." reads Psalms 51:7. Reading this against the backdrop of oregano's potent and broad anti-microbial properties, it is not difficult to imagine the line of thinking in that speculation.

More speculation exists about which specific oregano species contains the most potent therapeutic principles. Complications arise when trying to determine the real oregano. Sometimes this is due to very common errors in species name translation, while at other times

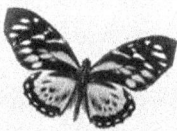

There is a place where primal passion is raised to the realms of ecstasy by the wings of love. And there is a place where guilt and shame and punishment reside. I can be a reminder that sexuality is good and true and beautiful. I can help heal the wounds from the shadow side of the mountain and I hope you will return to the light. Love is what gives wings to sex. Love asks permission. Love yourself and love others with ease and fun and harm to none.

it is a matter of misidentification. Yet, at other times, confusion is brought on by a hybrid of similar species. There is oregano, marjoram, Mexican oregano and so forth; all with varying amounts of biologically active ingredients. A study from Turkey reports: '...22 species of oregano of which the main species comprising oregano are Origanum majorana L., O. onites L., O. minutiflorum L., O. syrifimm L. and O. vulgare L. ssp. Hirtum.' This study further points out that 'of these species origanum majorana is a wild, native Turkish variety with a high Carvacrol content while the European oreganum majorana is cultivated on farms with relatively lower contents of Carvacrol.' Carvacrol is a well-studied phenol with known antiseptic properties, but only one of oregano's many constituents.

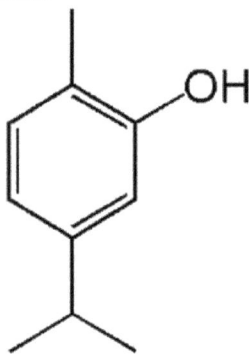

Carvacrol formula.

So, what are we to do with this? Consider the example with antibiotics. Initially a great drug in preventing infection, now a culprit in creating bacteria more potent than ever, which no antibiotic can touch. An antibiotic is one simple chemical compound, and life forms quickly mutate to survive it. Oregano may have retained her antimi- crobial potency throughout the ages due to a constantly shifting complex set of biologically active ingredients such as phenols, alkenes and alcohols. The nature of these ingredients also depends on various concentrations based on oregano species, richness of soil, weather influences, and processing techniques to which microbes cannot adjust.

Parts used: Leaves and flowers

Global summary:
Used to treat: arthritis, bursitis, analgesic, asthma (rubbed on chest), bad breath, colds, sore throats, gum infections, skin infections (acne, psoriasis, bites, bruises, burns, fungus, sores, canker sores, cold sores (HSV-1), shingles, head lice & scabies, parasites), irritable bowel disease, colic, diarrhea, digestive difficulties, cough, phlegm, bronchitis (inhaled), bladder infections, prostate difficulties, urinary tract difficulties, water retention, painful menstruation, sexually transmitted diseases and poor immunity.

Viral infections - examples: cold and flu viruses, warts, herpes, dengue fever, hepatitis, and chickenpox, all may respond to oil of oregano.

Parasite infestations - examples: ticks, giardia, hookworm, roundworm, ringworm, pinworm, flukes, malaria, sleeping sickness, schistosomiasis, tapeworm and other microbes, all may be completely destroyed or inhibited by oregano.

Bacterial infections - examples: cholera, salmonella, typhoid, diphteria, staph, tuberculosis, gonorrhea, bacterial meningitis, chlamidia.

Fungal infections - examples: candida albicans, athlete's foot, pityrosporum ovale (p. ovale) - or using its new name malassezia furfur, a fungi causing dandruff and seborrhea.

Used as a(n): antiseptic, antimicrobial (parasites, fungus, bacteria ,virus), antioxidant, anti-inflammatory, analgesic, agent to increase digestive juices (bile), cosmetic, antitussive (cough), immune stimulating, sedative, diuretic, diaphoretic, and tonic.

Due to the decade long overuse of antibiotics bacterial infections, such as gonorrhea, are becoming multi-drug resistant. The U.S. Center for Disease Control (CDC) released documentation in 2007 that we currently have only one class of anti-biotics left (Cephalosporins) in the 'arsenal' of pharmacological treatment options that are not currently resistant. But resistance is spreading making alternatives imperative. Penicillin, once a wonderdrug, is no longer used because it is largely ineffective. How long will the few remaining antibiotics last?

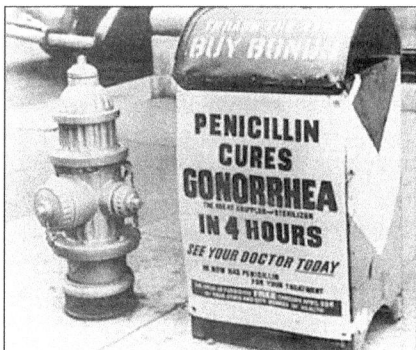

Courtesy: National Insitute of Health.

Cuba's traditional uses:
Rheumatoid arthritis, painful menstruation and urinary tract infections (UTI's).

Summary medicinal uses and prop-

erties supported by scientific studies:
Anti-parasitical (Chagas disease), antioxidant, anti-fungal, anti-bacterial (including several drug resistant strains), may reduce hyperglycemia, may support the immune system, and may be effective against leukemia (cancer).

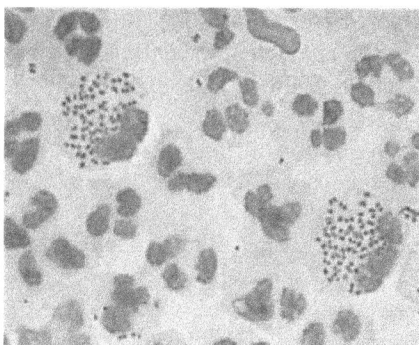

Gonorrhea Bacteria Collected by Neutrophils (White Blood Cells Destroying the Microbes)
Courtesy: CDC 1979

Brazil – Rio de Janeiro:
Oregano essential oil was used effectively in the laboratory against Trypanosoma cruzi, the parasite responsible for Chagas disease (T. cruzi infection) affecting humans and animals alike.[1] The CDC states that: "It is estimated that as many as 8 to 11 million people in Mexico, Central America, and South America have Chagas disease, most of whom do not know they are infected. If unrecognized and untreated, even silent infection is lifelong and can be life threatening."[2]

Bulgaria – Varna:
Scientists from the Department of Pharmacology and Biochemistry at the University of Medicine conducted studies following the model of traditional Bulgarian herbalists. Using a tea preparation of oregano to treat respiratory illness,

gastrointestinal problems and other inflammatory disorders, they discovered that tea of oregano has a high phenolic content as well as high anti-oxidant properties. This may account for its effectiveness for hundreds of years.[3]

China - Nanning:
Thymol and carvacrol were found by Chinese researchers to be the main compositions of the volatile oil of oregano.[4]

Italy - Bologna:
Veterinarians studied the effects of several essential oils including oil of oregano against candida fungal infections. They found it to have "maximum inhibitory activity"[5] of which the most active phenol component (acidic chemical compound with antiseptic properties) was carvacrol.

Mexico - Cuernavaca:
In this Mexican study scientists took samples from pediatric patients who were severely infected by gram-positive or gram-negative bacteria, which showed resistance to common antibiotics. These bacteria were then exposed in the laboratory to the commonly available essential oil of oregano, which recorded amongst the highest and broadest antibacterial activity.[6]

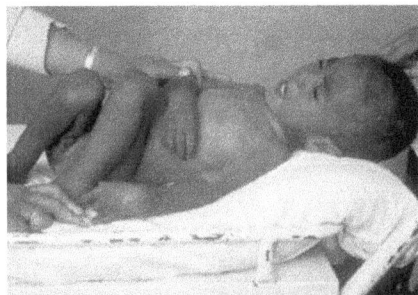

Courtesy: CDC 1970

Morocco - Errachidia:
Endocrinologists in Northern Africa examined the potential of a water-based extract of oregano as a therapeutic agent to treat hyperglycemia. They found in an animal model that the extract has the ability to reduce sugar levels without increasing the blood insulin concentrations.[7]

Russia:
This Russian study confirmed the antioxidant activity of extract of oregano.[8]

Spain - Madrid:
Scientists tested the antioxidant activity of oregano leaves extracted with a new process. This apparently environmentally friendly method called subcritical water extraction uses different temperatures. They determined that while all extract variants produced antioxidant capable solutions, those extracted at the highest temperature (200C°) offered the highest amount as well as the highest yield from the leaves.[9]

Switzerland - Dübendorf:
Good news for farmers from a recent study, which showed that adding oregano into the feed of growth-retarded pigs stimulates their immune system[10] thereby possibly allowing them to survive at a higher rate. This resulted in deeming oregano's therapeutic ability worthy of future exploration where immune improvement is required.

United States - Orlando:
Chemists at the University of Central Florida isolated several compounds from oregano. Studies showed that aristolochic acid I, and aristolochic acid II possessed cancer-fighting abilities, specifically against leukemia.[11]

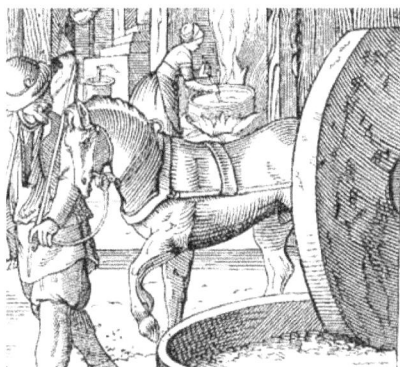

Oil making in the 16th century.
Engraved by J. Amman

PREPARATIONS:

A good essential oil of oregano is wild crafted and steam distilled. It usually takes many of the actual plants to make but a few drops of the essential oil. It is highly concentrated but with the diverse biologically active ingredients intact. The oil is not greasy, does not go rancid and has powerful antiseptic properties. When using the oil, use a steam distilled virgin oil (first pressing).

Oil of oregano internally: Take two to three drops daily of oil of oregano mixed with eight to twelve drops of a vegetable oil such as olive oil.

Oil of oregano externally: Apply directly to affected areas such as warts, inflammations, infections, and insect bites.

Dried herbs: use about 1gm twice a day.

To ensure you have an oregano plant with strong potential medicinal properties, buy only from a reputable purveyor, who uses wild, organic oregano plants, wild crafted, and with a relatively high concentration of Carvacrol.

Fresh herbs: Wild crafted and organic species of fresh oregano leaves and flowers tend to be strong in scent and flavor and can have a numbing effect upon contact with mucus membranes.

Tea: Pour a quarter liter of boiling water over two level teaspoons of the dried herb. Allow it to sit for about ten minutes, strain, inhale and drink to bring up phlegm, to treat and prevent arthritic flare-ups or use as a gargle to treat sore throats or oral infections.

Bath: Use but a few drops of the essential oil in baths. (Using too much may cause burning sensations, which water will not ease – to remedy burning sensations see below).

Unwanted Effects:

The essential oil of oregano may cause burning sensations upon contact with mucus membranes such as eyes, nose, mouth or genitals. This oil is not water-soluble and washing an affected area with water may only make it worse. When an irritation occurs use a vegetable oil to dilute. Usually the irritation will stop instantly.

Warning:

As of 1988, 'the German Commission E' considered oregano an unapproved drug due to the lack of documented efficacy at that time.

Possible interaction with drugs:

Currently no data is available indicating possible drug interactions.

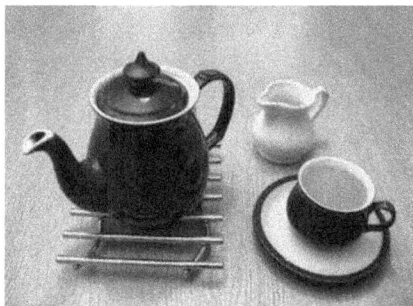

Courtesy: Vanderdecken

Amharic: Oregano
Dutch: Wilde Marjolein
French: Origan sauvage
German: Oregano
Hebrew: Oregano
Hindi: Sathra
Homeopathic: Origanum vulgare
(Orig-v.)
Italian: Origano
Korean: Oregano
Latin: Origanum vulgare
Russian: Dushitsa
Spanish: Orégano

1 Santoro GF, das Graças Cardoso M, Guimarães LG, Salgado AP, Menna-Barreto RF, Soares MJ. *Effect of oregano (Origanum vulgare L.) and thyme (Thymus vulgaris L.) essential oils on Trypanosoma cruzi (Protozoa: Kinetoplastida) growth and ultrastructure.* Laboratório de Biologia Celular de Microrganismos, Departamento de Ultra-estrutura e Biologia Celular, Instituto Oswaldo Cruz/FIOCRUZ, Avenida Brasil 4365 Manguinhos, 21040-900, Rio de Janeiro, Rio de Janeiro, Brazil. Parasitol Res. 2007 Mar;100(4):783-90.

2 http://www.cdc.gov/ncidod/dpd/parasites/chagasdisease/factsht_chagas_disease.htm

3 Ivanova D, Gerova D, Chervenkov T, Yankova T. *Polyphenols and antioxidant capacity of Bulgarian medicinal plants.* Department of Pharmacology and Biochemistry, University of Medicine Varna, 55 Marin Drinov Street, 9002 Varna, Bulgaria. J Ethnopharmacol. 2005 Jan 4;96(1-2):145-50.

4 Tian H, Lai DM. *Analysis on the volatile oil in Origanum vulgare.* Guangxi College of TCM, Nanning 530001, China. Zhong Yao Cai. 2006 Sep;29(9):920-1.

5 Tampieri MP, Galuppi R, Macchioni F, Carelle MS, Falcioni L, Cioni PL, Morelli I. *The inhibition of Candida albicans by selected essential oils and their major components.* Dipartimento di Sanità Pubblica Veterinaria e Patologia Animale, Università di Bologna, Italy. Mycopathologia. 2005 Apr;159(3):339-45.

6 Hersch-Martínez P, Leaños-Miranda BE, Solórzano-Santos F. *Antibacterial effects of commercial essential oils over locally prevalent pathogenic strains in Mexico.* Proyecto Actores Sociales de la Flora Medicinal en México, Instituto Nacional de Antropología e Historia, Matamoros 14, Acapantzingo, Cuernavaca, Morelos 62440, Mexico. Fitoterapia. 2005 Jul;76(5):453-7.

7 Lemhadri A, Zeggwagh NA, Maghrani M, Jouad H, Eddouks M. *Anti-hyperglycaemic activity of the aqueous extract of Origanum vulgare growing wild in Tafilalet region.* Laboratory of Endocrinian Physiology, F.S.T.E. Boutalamine and Pharmacology, UFR PNPE, BP 21, Errachidia 52000, Morocco. J Ethnopharmacol. 2004 Jun;92(2-3):251-6.

8 Ryzhikov MA, Ryzhikova VO. *Application of chemiluminescent methods for analysis of the antioxidant activity of herbal extracts.* Vopr Pitan. 2006;75(2):22-6.

9 Rodríguez-Meizoso I, Marin FR, Herrero M, Señorans FJ, Reglero G, Cifuentes A, Ibáñez E. *Subcritical water extraction of nutraceuticals with antioxidant activity from oregano. Chemical and functional characterization.* Departamento de Caracterización de Alimentos, Instituto de Fermentaciones Industriales (CSIC), Juan de la Cierva 3, 28006 Madrid, Spain. J Pharm Biomed Anal. 2006 Aug 28;41(5):1560-5.

10 Walter BM, Bilkei G. *Immunostimulatory effect of dietary oregano etheric oils on lymphocytes from growth-retarded, low-weight growing-finishing pigs and productivity.* Bilkei Consulting, Raubbühlstrasse 4, 8600 Dübendorf, Switzerland. Tijdschr Diergeneeskd. 2004 Mar 15;129(6):178-81.

11 Goun E, Cunningham G, Solodnikov S, Krasnykh O, Miles H. *Antithrombin activity of some constituents from Origanum vulgare.* Department of Chemistry, University of Central Florida, Orlando, FL 32816, USA. Fitoterapia. 2002 Dec;73(7-8):692-4.

Growth: Oregano is a perennial plant that can reach up to 2 feet in height about 1 foot in width.

Native to: Mediterranean but can be grown is a variety of climates.

How to grow oregano: It is very easy to grow oregano. Obtain organic seeds and sprinkle them directly onto loose dry soil. If the soil is porous enough to allow the seeds to be slightly swallowed you don't need to cover them with a very thin layer of topsoil. Use a spray bottle and apply a mist of water until the topsoil layer and the seeds are covered with a bit of water. Keep the soil slightly moist and in about a week or two you will see the tiny sprout rising from the soil. Allow them to form roots and a few leafs and grow until there are about three inches in height and than transplant them in clusters into their new home, a pot will do, or straight into the garden. Find a spot with good sun and well-drained soil and plant them a little less that a foot apart. Once the oregano plant are established in your garden they can handle relative dry conditions but not for prolonged periods of time. If you have a dry spell you can water the plants slightly about once a week. Increase leaf abundance, taste and oil content by removing the flowers from their stems as soon as they appear.

Time to seed: Seed directly into the garden soil in spring after the last frost has passed. You can start in seedbeds or pots inside weeks before.

Sun: Full sun.

Zone: 4 – 9

Soil: Loose, well drained, organic garden soil. No fertilizer needed, a curious fact, if you do fertilize, you will diminish oil of oregano intensity.

Harvest: You can begin harvesting oregano as soon as the plant has established several stems with multiple sets of leaves. The oil of oregano is more easily accessible in fresh leaves in the morning hours when the leaves pores are still more open than later in the day when the sun gets brighter.

   To dry individually picked leaves, spread them out on a dry, clean and breathable surface. Keep them in a ventilated room until dry. You can also cut entire stems with leafs attached and hang them upside down in the same place until dry, and than remove them from the stem.

   When the plant begins to wither in late fall or early winter cut the stems down to their base and cover the stumps with mulch to protect them from the winter environment. They will return for a couple of years before re-seeding is necessary.

Attracts friends: Bees, butterflies and other pollinating animals.

Storage: Fresh oregano kept in a small plastic bag and refrigerated or frozen will prolong their properties of taste and therapeutics.

ROSMARINUS
OFFICINALIS

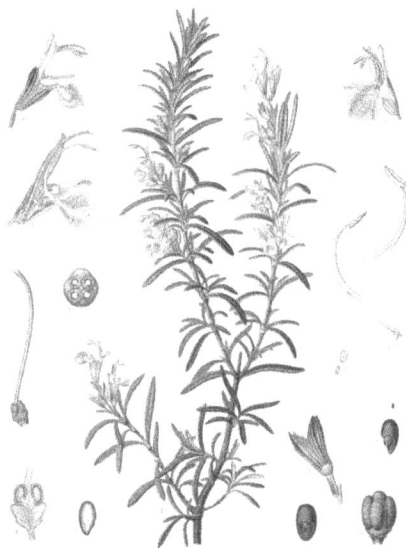

Köhler's Medicinal Plants 1887

Rosemary

I have the
potential to
nurture and
support you.

Rosemary's reputation for curing baldness, headaches and enhancing memory is so ancient that the English refer to it as 'Old Man'. In Shakespeare's Hamlet, Ophelia said: "There's rosemary, that's for remembrance." The Latin name for rosemary is Rosmarinus, 'ros', meaning dew, and 'marinus' of the sea. Christian's named her 'the rose of Mary,' from a tale of Mary laying her cloak over the rosemary plant then retrieving it to reveal blue flowers where there had been none.

The aromatic and hardy rosemary plant originally claimed home around the Mediterranean, but nowadays can be found almost anywhere in the world where the climate and ground allows it. It is very easy to cultivate and drought-resistant. You can use clippings from a mature plant, place them

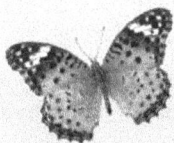

My spirit has a seductive way of relaxing your liver and gall and like the tight tension of a muscle set free by a burst of spontaneous laughter juices may flow more freely and mix in the right amounts with the foods you have eaten. It will flow more freely through you, making it easier to assimilate, digest and eliminate. But I must warn you; this may result in feeling happy and being nurtured, feeling safe and relaxed.

in a glass of water until roots appear, and plant in a bright and sunny spot. You will quickly find fresh rosemary at your fingertips.

Parts used: Fresh or dried leaves picked while flowering.

Global summary:
Used to treat: colds, flu, weakened liver and gall bladder (for example, low bile production), gastro-intestinal spasms, flatulence, poor circulation, rheumatism, skin inflammation, difficulty menstruating, wounds, pain, bad breath, balding, dandruff, loss of appetite, and the circulatory, nervous and digestive systems.
Used as a(n): astringent, diaphoretic, analgesic, hepa-protector (liver protector), choleretic (increases bile production), skin tonic, antispasmodic, menstruation facilitator, carminative (reduces flatulence), anti ager, and as a hair tonic.

Cuba's traditional uses:
Romero belongs to the goddess of the sea, Yemaya. Yerberos use it to cure headaches, rheumatism, and as an alcohol rub to treat generalized muscular pain.

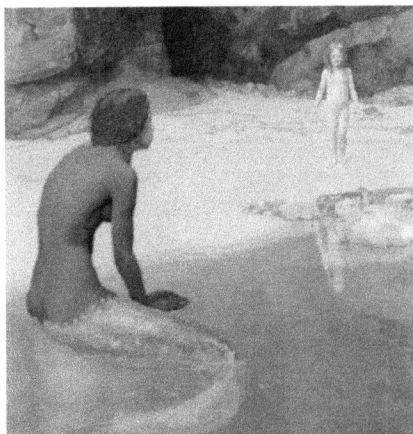
Courtesy: John Collier (pic. altered) 1899

Summary medicinal uses and properties supported by scientific studies:
Anti-microbial (bacteria, fungi), dyspepsia (digestive complaints), promotes circulation, radio protective, may be effective in skin cancer tumor prevention, may prevent other kinds of tumors, anti-inflammatory, may help in the prevention and treatment of diabetic, cardiovascular, and other neurodegenerative diseases.

China - Harbin:
Scientists confirmed the anti-microbial activity of the essential oil of rosemary against a variety of bacterial and fungal pathogens including those of Staphylococcus epidermidis, Escherichia coli and Candida albicans.[1]

Cuba's clinical uses:
An infusion of rosemary leaves is used in Cuba to treat liver and gall bladder complaints, and is also used to reduce spasms due to gas, as well as flatulence itself. Furthermore, it is also used as a tonic for hair.

German Commission E:
Approved for: "Internal: Dyspeptic complaints. External: Supportive therapy for rheumatic diseases, circulatory problems."

India - Jaipur:
In this controlled study researchers uncovered rosemary's ability to protect laboratory animals from the damage of ionizing radiation.[2]

India - Jaipur:
A mouse model was used to determine the anti-tumor properties of rosemary in the case of chemically induced skin cancer formation. Those mice fed 1gm/kg

of rosemary extract by weight sustained an average of approximately 50% reduction of tumor formation when compared to the untreated control group.[3]

Taiwan - Taichung Hsien:

Scientists from this island nation conducted a set of experiments using a super critical fluid extraction technique and identified several biologically active constituents from rosemary determining that it: "…can be considered an herbal anti-inflammatory and anti-tumor agent."[4]

Taiwan - Taichung Hsien:

In another experiment from the same University scientists concluded that: "… rosemary is an excellent multifunctional therapeutic herb; by looking at its potentially potent antiglycative bioactivity, it may become a good adjuvant medicine for the prevention and treatment of diabetic, cardiovascular, and other neurodegenerative diseases."[5]

Both tradition and science agree rosemary is an herb for many occasions. In Santeria rosemary belongs to the realm of the goddess of the sea. Does the mystery of the deep hold the secret to understanding why this herb is so versatile, will Yemaya reveal the secret?

PREPARATIONS:

Rosemary tea: Pour one liter of boiling water over five grams of rosemary leaves. Drink two cups of the tea throughout the day as a tonic.

Rosemary wine: In German Folk medicine Rosemary wine is used as a cardio, nervous system and digestive tonic. Cut approximately 20-25gm rosemary leaves (or one handful fresh rosemary leaves or two to three tablespoons of dried rosemary leaves) and macerate in one liter of white wine for two to five days. During maceration, agitate the fluid occasionally. Upon completion of maceration run the fluid through a strainer, compost the plant matter and store the liquid in a dark bottle protecting it from sunlight. Take in small quantities.

Topical hair and dandruff treatment: An infusion of rosemary flowers and leaves combined with borax, a natural mineral salt with its own antifungal properties applied to the scalp as a treatment for dandruff. Use 1 cup of dried rosemary leaves, 1 liter of boiling water and a tablespoon of borax. Let it steep over night. Strain it and use as a final rinse after showering.

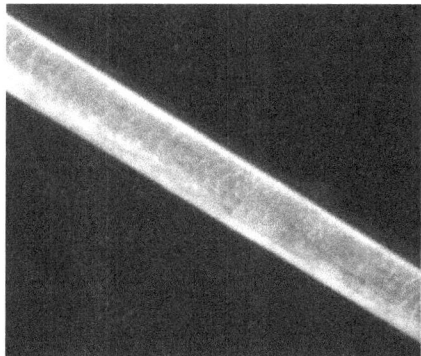

The Human Hair Magnified.
Courtesy: Jan Homann.

Rosemary essential oils:

These oils are very concentrated and should be used with caution. As always with essential oils, test on a small area of skin for allergic reactions. Avoid contact with mucus membranes. If you have an accidental contact do not use water. Essential oils are not water-soluble and tend to only spread the oil and intensify sensations. Use any vegetable oil to dilute the essential oil, and the burning sensations should quickly subside.

Unwanted Effects:

Due to its stimulating effect it may be more difficult to go to sleep at night. Experiment by drinking the infusion during the day only. Contact allergies have been observed on rare occasions.

WARNING:

Do not use rosemary during pregnancy. Rosemary, especially the essential oil, may induce uterine contractions. It has been reported that very large quantities of rosemary oil have brought on abortions. Furthermore, over doses of essential oil of rosemary ingestion have been reported to cause seizures, kidney failure and death.

Possible interaction with drugs:

There is currently no data available indicating possible drug interactions.

Amharic: Azmarina
Dutch: Rozemarijn
French: Romarin
German: Rosmarin
Hebrew: Rozmarin
Hindi: Rusmari
Homeopathic:Rosmarinus officinalis
(Rosm.)
Italian: Rosmarino
Korean: Rojumeri
Latin: Rosemarinus officinalis
Russian: Rozmarin
Spanish: Rosmario
Tigrinya: Azmarina

1 Fu Y, Zu Y, Chen L, Shi X, Wang Z, Sun S, Efferth T. *Antimicrobial activity of clove and rosemary essential oils alone and in combination.* Key Laboratory of Forest Plant Ecology, Ministry of Education, Northeast Forestry University, Harbin 150040, P. R. China. Phytother Res. 2007 Jun 11.

2 Soyal D, Jindal A, Singh I, Goyal PK. *Modulation of radiation-induced biochemical alterations in mice by rosemary (Rosemarinus officinalis) extract.* Radiation and Cancer Biology Laboratory, Department of Zoology, University of Rajasthan, Jaipur 302004, India. Phytomedicine. 2007 Oct;14(10):701-5.

3 Sancheti G, Goyal P. *Modulatory influence of Rosemarinus officinalis on DMBA-induced mouse skin tumorigenesis.* Radiation and Cancer Biology Lab, Dept Zoology, University of Rajasthan, Jaipur, 302 004 India. garimasancheti@ rediffmailcom Asian Pac J Cancer Prev. 2006 Apr-Jun;7(2):331-5.

4 Peng CH, Su JD, Chyau CC, Sung TY, Ho SS, Peng CC, Peng RY. *Supercritical fluid extracts of rosemary leaves exhibit potent anti-inflammation and anti-tumor effects.* Division of Basic Medical Science, Hungkuang University, No 34, Chung Chie Rd, Shalu County, Taichung Hsien, 43302, Taiwan. Biosci Biotechnol Biochem. 2007 Sep;71(9):2223-32.

5 Hsieh CL, Peng CH, Chyau CC, Lin YC, Wang HE, Peng RY. *Low-density lipoprotein, collagen, and thrombin models reveal that Rosemarinus officinalis L. exhibits potent antiglycative effects.* Department of Food and Nutrition, Research Institute of Biotechnology, and Division of Basic Medical Sciences, Hung-Kuang University, No. 34 Chung-Chie Road, Shalu County, Taichung Hsien, Taiwan. J Agric Food Chem. 2007 Apr 18;55(8):2884-91.

Growth: In a frost-free area rosemary is hardy perennial plant can grow as a plant and as a shrub between 3 – 6 feet.

Native to: Most environments adjacent to the Mediterranean Sea.

How to grow rosemary: While rosemary can be grown from seed it is easier to make cuttings of about 3 – 6 inches long from fresh shoots of an established plant. Make several of the cuttings ideally in late spring when the plant is full of growing energy. Brush the leaves off the lower part of the stem and place them in a glass of water and place it on a warm windowsill until you have about an inch or more of roots. Or place the cleared stem directly into a small container containing your wet soil. Keep the plant in a sunny, sheltered location and keep the soil moist until you feel them rooted. Root growth may take up to two months. You can enhance your success rate by using an organic rooting enzyme and by dipping the leaf free stem about a ¼ inch deep into it and than into the wet soil.

Time to grow: Best when making cuttings in late spring or prior to flowering.

Sun: Full sun and some partial shade is o.k.

Zone: 6 - 10

Soil: Organic, well-drained normal garden soil will do fine. Once established, these plants are quite drought tolerant. No fertilizer required.

Harvest: Allow the plant to reach a couple of feet in height and you are ready to harvest. You can cut off a few new branches and pull the leaves off against their growing direction. Use the leaves fresh for you culinary or medicinal needs, freeze fresh or dry them as you desire. The plant will recover quickly and provide you with more leaves to work with.

Attracts friends: Hovering Syrphid flies help pollinate and Syrphid fly larvae will eat aphids and other soft bodies garden pests. They do not sting even if they look wasp like to some.

Environmental benefits: Protects from garden pests such as Carrot flies, Bean Beetles and Cabbage Moths

Storage: Hang the stems with their leaves in place upside down in a dark, dry and airy room. When dry peel the off the stem and keep them stored in a dry container until you need them.

CURCUMA
LONGA

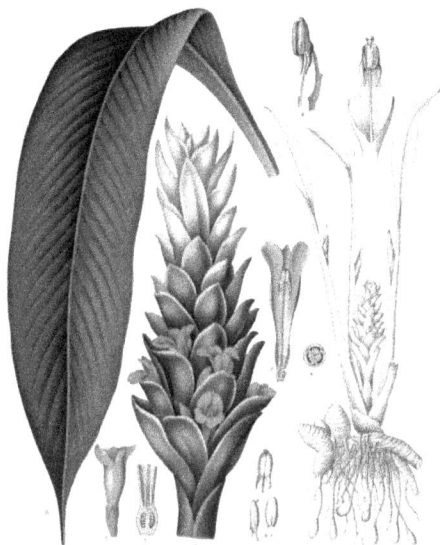

Köhler's Medicinal Plants 1887

Turmeric

I am a boundary dweller and a bridge amidst the worlds. I live in between, where one thing begins, and another ends.

The origin of turmeric is not exactly known. However, ancient records place it anywhere from China to Southeast Asia where it was once used to color clothing and even lighten darker skin complexions. Now modern science has discovered turmeric. The U.S. National Library currently has more than 700 published scientific studies listed where turmeric or components thereof are being probed and examined. These scientists are only catching up with turmeric's long-documented history as an ancient spice and medicine.

The plant prefers a tropical environment with plenty of rain. Today, it is cultivated as a major crop in the tropical regions of China, India, Indonesia and Thailand, turmeric is also found in tropical African regions such as Madagascar. It has a

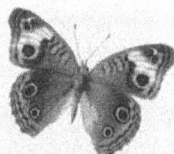

I reside at the edge where you create a sacred space by your desire and belief, and where life responds to fill the void therein accordingly. You can trust yourself to learn, to know, of what is good for you. Let this knowledge rise to nurture and support you in digesting, absorbing and eliminating what life brings your way.

proven track record as a flavorful spice and safe and effective medicinal herb. In fact, with scientific evidence so convincing multi-national pharmaceutical corporations are trying (as in the case with neem) to patent turmeric. To date, the United States Patent Office has rejected these corporations' attempts to control this ancient herbal spice. We can still access strong and safe medicine without having to spend a fortune on a patent-controlled monopoly of the pharmaceutical industry.

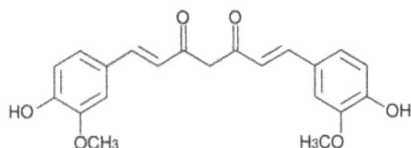

**Curcumin as Functional Group - Ketone.
Courtesy: Mysid**

Parts used: The rhizome (usually ground into a fine powder) and tubers.

Global summary:
Used to treat: amenorrhoea (absence of menstrual period), dysmenorrhoea (difficult menstruation or painful menstruation), female facial hair, diarrhea, epilepsy, pain, skin diseases, parasites, urinary calculi (kidney stones), gallbladder stones, liver diseases (hepatitis), jaundice, diabetes, digestive difficulties (dyspepsia), Crohn's-disease, high stomach acidity, oxidative stress, peptic ulcers, slow memory function, and skin diseases such as scabies.

Used as a(n): antioxidant, anti-carcinogenic (prevention and treatment), anti-inflammatory and painkiller (especially in arthritis and rheumatoid arthritis), blood thinner, cataract prevention, breast milk stimulator, memory enhancer, mild diuretic (reduces blood pressure), liver

and kidney protector, stimulator of bile flow (thereby may prevent cholesterol-based gallbladder stone formation and assist in their elimination), digestive fluids promoter and gas reducer, immunomodulator, antiviral, antibacterial, and antifungal.

Summary medicinal uses and properties supported by scientific studies 2004-2007:
Anti-parasitical (schistosomiasis); anti-bacterial; pulmonary protective; digestive difficulties; prevents relapse in cases of ulcerative colitis; Crohn's disease; stomach ulcers; cancer preventative; cancer treatment; promoter of wound-healing and diabetes. A therapeutic agent in Alzheimer's, Parkinson disease, cardio-vascular disease, pulmonary disease, arthritis, adenomatous polyposis (multiple polyps in the large intestines – precursor to colon cancer), inflammatory bowel disease (IBS), ulcerative colitis (colon inflammation with ulcers), arthritis, atherosclerosis, pancreatitis, psoriasis, chronic anterior and uveitis (inflammation of the middle layer of the eye). Anti-inflammatory, immune modulator, allergies, atherosclerosis, heart disease, and diabetes.

Egypt - Cairo:
Scientists compared the effectiveness of turmeric and praziquantel, the paharmacological treatment of choice, in destroying the parasite schitosomiasis. They discovered that turmeric was better at lowering parasitical egg counts while praziquantel was better able to reduce actual worm presence.[1]

England - London:
Scientists examined the antibacterial properties of the extract against Helico-

bacter pylori (the bacteria held responsible for contributing to stomach ulcers) and found that of the 25 plants tested turmeric had the strongest antibacterial properties. It not only destroyed the bacteria, it also prevented it from attaching to the stomach walls, which scientists suggested could provide an effective alternative to antibiotic resistant strains of the microbe.[2]

France – Vandoeuvre-Lès-Nancy

Based on the evidence of numerous laboratory and animal trials these scientists contend "...that curcumin plays a protective role in chronic obstructive pulmonary disease, acute lung injury, acute respiratory distress syndrome, and allergic asthma, its therapeutic action being on the prevention or modulation of inflammation and oxidative stress." Furthermore, and based on the substance of these studies, "these scientists suggest the beginning of clinical trials using turmeric to treat human patients with a variety of chronic and acute lung disorders."[3]

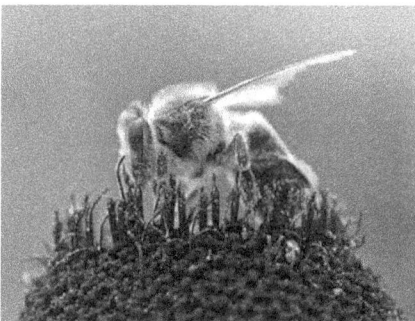

Pollen Collecting Bee. Courtesy: Jon Sullivan

German Commission E:

Turmeric was approved in the treatment of digestive difficulties with a dose range of 1.5 – 3gm daily.

Japan – Hamamatsu:

In this double-blind randomized placebo controlled human study scientists examined turmeric's ability to assist patients with a history of dormant ulcerative colitis from relapsing. They concluded that curcumin, an active ingredient in turmeric, seemed to be a safe medication for maintaining remission from ulcerative colitis.[4]

Thailand – Bangkok:

In a study conducted in Thailand patients with peptic ulcers were given 2 capsules filled with turmeric (300 mg each) orally, 5 times daily. The result after 4 weeks of treatment showed that ulcers were absent in 48% of the cases treated with turmeric.[5]

United States – Dallas:

In this meta-study scientists give an overview of decades of scientific studies on turmeric. They summarize a long list of turmeric's potential therapeutic properties: cancer and diabetic preventative, cancer treatment, promoter of wound-healing, therapeutic agent in Alzheimer's, Parkinson's, cardio-vascular, and pulmonary disease, arthritis, adenomatous polyposis (multiple polyps in the large intestines – precursor to colon cancer), inflammatory bowel disease (IBS), ulcerative colitis (colon inflammation with ulcers), atherosclerosis, pancreatitis, psoriasis, chronic anterior and uveitis (inflammation of the middle layer of the eye).[6]

United States – Houston:

Research over the past five decades, time-proven records from other traditions, and numerous case studies have indicated that turmeric can prevent and treat some forms of cancer. Turmeric has the ability to diminish the creation, production and spread of a wide variety of tumor cells.[7]

United States - Houston:
A University of Texas M. D. Anderson Cancer Center study confirms time-proven traditional knowledge boasting turmeric's anti-inflammatory properties. In addition, they discovered that turmeric modulates the immune system by activating natural killer cells. When used in low doses, turmeric reduces the body's tendency to produce pro-inflammatory cytokines by enhancing antibody response. In cases of asthma, arthritis, allergies, atherosclerosis, heart disease, Alzheimer's disease, diabetes, and cancer researchers suggest that curcumin's (yellow-orange colored part of turmeric) reported beneficial effects may be related to this immune modulating property.[8]

If this is indeed the case what other immune deficiencies can benefit from turmeric in their lives?

United States - Houston:
In another study from the Cancer Center scientists stated that one of the problems with turmeric is the low bioavailability due to rapid elimination and poor absorption. But, they also realized that even while they are trying to overcome this hurdle turmeric, in its current bioavailability, is able to produce therapeutic effects in cases of different diseases such as "…cancer, cardiovascular diseases, diabetes, arthritis, neurological diseases and Crohn's disease…"[9]

United States - Houston:
Another study focused on the combined results of the past decades of scientific study using turmeric as a means to enhance immunity by the activation of '… T cells, B cells, macrophages, neutrophils, natural killer cells, and dendritic cells…on one hand and on the other to be able to reduce pro-inflammatory cytokines (chemical messengers inducing inflammation).'

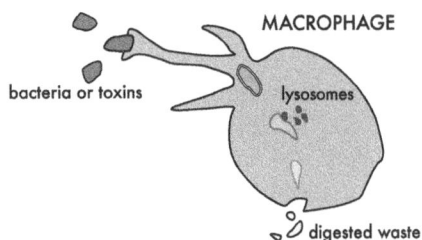

An immune system cell, called a macrophage, engulfs a bacteria or toxins. A lysosome (an organelle/part of the macrophage) merges with the engulfment and injects acidic (pH 4.5) digestive enzymes and oxidizing hydrogen peroxide into the 'engulfed food,' which is destroyed and expelled as 'harmless' particles.

United States - San Francisco:
Scientists at the University of California determined in this study that turmeric also has potent anti-inflammatory properties.[10]

W.H.O. Monographs on selected Medicinal Plants:
"Uses supported by clinical data: The principal use of Rhizoma Curcumae Longae is for the treatment of acid, flatulent, or atonic dyspepsia."

Uses described in pharmacopoeias and in traditional systems of medicine: "Treatment of peptic ulcers, and pain and inflammation due to rheumatoid arthritis and of amenorrhoea, dysmenorrhoea, diarrhoea, epilepsy, pain, and skin diseases."

PREPARATIONS:

Dried herb: Suggested dose for prevention and treatment is 1 gm twice a day. Human clinical trials are indicated safe for doses up to 12 gm/day.[11] Also available as a tincture, extract, powder, paste, ointment, essential oil, oil, lotion, and as an inhalant depending in which country you live. Good quality turmeric should have a red-orange colored look to it.

WARNING:

Allergic contact dermatitis (inflammation of the skin) has been noted in some people. Liver toxicity has been reported with the use of the spice and alcohol extracts in experiments with mice.[12]

Use caution with the use of essential oils. Always test on a small portion of skin before using them to avoid contact dermatitis.

In the case of gallbladder stones consult a healthcare professional. A sudden increase in bile flow may cause pains and stone movement and, depending on the size of the stone(s), may contribute to significant pain and bile duct obstruction.

Do not use during pregnancies. Studies have suggested - as do the uses from other countries where turmeric is used to regulate menstruations - that turmeric stimulates activity of the uterus and may cause abortion.

Possible interaction with drugs:

Turmeric may protect against the formation of stomach ulcers produced by many non-steroidal anti-inflammatory drugs (NSAID's) and other pharmaceutical medication or chemical irritants.

Saudi Arabia - Riyadh:

Indocin is a NSAID commonly prescribed to treat swelling and pains due to arthritis. A common side effect is stomach ulcers. Reserpine, an anti-psychotic drug, also commonly produces stomach ulcers. In 1990, scientists from King Saud University discovered that turmeric extract given to rats at the dose of 500mg/kg was enough to: "...produce significant anti-ulcerogenic activity."[13]

South Korea:

These scientists conducted further experiments to determine the exact physiological mechanism of how turmeric prevents the formation of stomach ulcers and found that "the extract from C. longa specifically inhibits gastric acid secretion by blocking H(2) histamine receptors in a competitive manner."[14]

Amharic: Ird
Dutch: Geelwortel
French: Curcuma
German: Gelbwurzel, Kurkuma
Hebrew: Kurkum
Hindi: Haldi
Homeopathic: Curcuma longa (Curc.)
Italian: Curcuma
Korean: Tumerik
Latin: Curcuma longa
Russian: Kurkuma
Sanskrit: Haridraa
Spanish: Rhizome de curcuma
Swahili: Manjano
Tirinya: Irdi

1 El-Ansary AK, Ahmed SA, Aly SA. *Antischistosomal and liver protective effects of Curcuma longa extract in Schistosoma mansoni infected mice.* Medicinal Chemistry Department, National Research Centre, Dokki, Cairo, Egypt. Indian J Exp Biol. 2007 Sep;45(9):791-801.

2 O'Mahony R, Al-Khtheeri H, Weerasekera D, Fernando N, Vaira D, Holton J, Basset C. *Bactericidal and anti-adhesive properties of culinary and medicinal plants against Helicobacter pylori.* Centre for Infectious Diseases and International

Health, Royal Free and University College London Medical School, Windeyer Building, 46 Cleveland Street, London, W1P 6DB, United Kingdom. World J Gastroenterol. 2005 Dec 21;11(47):7499-507.

3 Venkatesan N, Punithavathi D, Babu M. *Protection from acute and chronic lung diseases by curcumin*. Faculte de Medecine, UMR-7561, CNRS UHP, Vandoeuvre lès Nancy, France. vnar12@yahoo.com Adv Exp Med Biol. 2007;595:379-405.

4 Hanai H, Iida T, Takeuchi K, Watanabe F, Maruyama Y, Andoh A, Tsujikawa T, Fujiyama Y, Mitsuyama K, Sata M, Yamada M, Iwaoka Y, Kanke K, Hiraishi H, Hirayama K, Arai H, Yoshii S, Uchijima M, Nagata T, Koide Y. *Curcumin maintenance therapy for ulcerative colitis: randomized, multicenter, double-blind, placebo-controlled trial*. Department of Endoscopic and Photodynamic Medicine, Hamamatsu University School of Medicine, and Center for Gastroenterology, Hamamatsu South Hospital, Hamamatsu, Japan. Clin Gastroenterol Hepatol. 2006 Dec;4(12):1502-6.

5 Prucksunand C, Indrasukhsri B, Leethochawalit M, Hungspreugs K. *Phase II clinical trial on effect of the long turmeric (Curcuma longa Linn) on healing of peptic ulcer*. Department of Pharmacology, Faculty of Medicine, Siriraj Hospital, Mahidol University, Bangkok, Thailand. Southeast Asian J Trop Med Public Health. 2001 Mar;32(1):208-15.

6 Goel A, Kunnumakkara AB, Aggarwal BB. Curcumin as "Curecumin": *From kitchen to clinic*. Gastrointestinal Cancer Research Laboratory, Department of Internal Medicine, Charles A. Sammons Cancer Center and Baylor Research Institute, Baylor University Medical Center, Dallas, TX, United States. Biochem Pharmacol. 2007 Aug 19.

7 Aggarwal BB, Kumar A, Bharti AC. *Anticancer potential of curcumin: preclinical and clinical studies*. Cytokine Research Section, Department of Bioimmunotherapy, University of Texas M. D. Anderson Cancer Center, 1515 Holcombe Boulevard, Box 143, Houston, TX, USA. Anticancer Research. 2003 Jan-Feb;23(1A):363-98.

8 Jagetia GC, Aggarwal BB. *"Spicing up" of the immune system by curcumin*. Cytokine Research Laboratory, Department of Experimental Therapeutics, The University of Texas M. D. Anderson Cancer Center, Houston, Texas, USA. J Clin Immunol. 2007 Jan;27(1):19-35.

9 Anand P, Kunnumakkara AB, Newman RA, Aggarwal BB. *Bioavailability of Curcumin: Problems and Promises*. Cytokine Research Laboratory and Pharmaceutical Development Center, Department of Experimental Therapeutics, The University of Texas M. D. Anderson Cancer Center, Houston, Texas 77030 aggarwal@mdanderson.org Mol Pharm. 2007 Nov 14.

10 Chainani-Wu N. *Safety and anti-inflammatory activity of curcumin: a component of tumeric (Curcuma longa)*. Department of Stomatology, University of California, San Francisco, CA 94143-0658, USA. J Altern Complement Med. 2003 Feb;9(1):161-8.

11 Anand P, Kunnumakkara AB, Newman RA, Aggarwal BB. *Bioavailability of Curcumin: Problems and Promises*. Cytokine Research Laboratory and Pharmaceutical Development Center, Department of Experimental Therapeutics, The University of Texas M. D. Anderson Cancer Center, Houston, Texas 77030 aggarwal@mdanderson.org Mol Pharm. 2007 Nov 14.

12 Kandarkar SV, Sawant SS, Ingle AD, Deshpande SS, Maru GB. *Subchronic oral hepatotoxicity of turmeric in mice--histopathological and ultrastructural studies*. Cell Biology Division, Tata Memorial Centre, Mumbai, India. Indian J Exp Biol. 1998 Jul;36(7):675-9.

13 Rafatullah S, Tariq M, Al-Yahya MA, Mossa JS, Ageel AM. *Evaluation of turmeric (Curcuma longa) for gastric and duodenal antiulcer activity in rats*. Medicinal, Aromatic and Poisonous Plants Research Center, College of Pharmacy, King Saud University, Riyadh, Saudi Arabia. J Ethnopharmacol. 1990 Apr;29(1):25-34.

14 Kim DC, Kim SH, Choi BH, Baek NI, Kim D, Kim MJ, Kim KT. *Curcuma longa extract protects against gastric ulcers by blocking H2 histamine receptors*. Division of Molecular and Life Science, SBD-NCRC, Pohang University of Science and Technology, South Korea. Biol Pharm Bull. 2005 Dec;28(12):2220-4.

Growth: Turmeric is a perennial plant that, depending on species grows on average from 3 to about 4 feet in height.

Native to: Tropical Southern Asia but is grown in many similar climates around the globe.

How to grow turmeric: The plant is propagated by dividing the rhizomes and than planting them in a new location. The transplant can be quick and easy in humid, tropical soil and climate while in other location it may take a bit more care. In a colder climate it can also be grown entirely on the inside and still produce potent turmeric.

Find some organic turmeric rhizomes, of the kind you like to grow, at a market or grower and pick several pieces that are shiny, fat in appearance, containing several fingers and do not have cracked or chapped dry skin.

To grow the plant in a 3 gallon pot choose a few pieces and place them into the soil covered with about a half an inch of soil. Keep the soil moist but not soaking wet. Cover with a plastic bag and keep in the dark. When applying water check to see which of the rhizomes are beginning to sprout. Weed out the rest and place the pot with the plant in a warm place with indirect but good light.

Time to grow: In the tropics anytime. In cooler climates you can give the plant a head start inside in pots or wait until the last frost has passed and plant straight into the soil. Temperature zone 8-11 can be planted straight into the soil. Move the plants inside before the first frost appears. Let the leaves wither and cut them down to the root and allow the plant to hibernate through the winter. Just a little of moisture occasionally is all the care required. Bring them out again next spring.

Sun: Full sun to partial shade.

Zone: 10 – 12

Soil: Well drained, loose, rich organic soil.

Harvest: It takes about 5 to 6 month to produce new rhizome growth. You can see the new growth as it will creep sideway right at the edge of soil and air. Harvest anytime after the plant has been established. In case of a cooler climate harvest part of the rhizomes as you prep the rest of plant for winter.

Attracts friends: The plant will produce flowers after a few growing cycles, usually between 2 to four years. The flowers attract bees, butterflies and hummingbirds.

Environmental benefits: Ants do not like to cross-powdered turmeric.

Storage: Ground turmeric powder should be kept in a tight, dry container stored in a dark place.

PLANT HARDINESS ZONE SCALE

The plant hardiness zone scale is not an exact mechanism to predict if a plant will grow there. Other factors such as altitude, soil types, wind conditions, rain fall patterns, micro-climates, humidity or the lack of it might be helpful to take into consideration. It is always helpful to get advise from local gardeners who have some experience with the type of plant you like to grow.

Plant Hardiness Zones for North America, China and Northern Europe are rated on a scale from 1 through 11. South America 1 through 13 and Africa 7 through 13. Zone 1 represents the approximate average coldest temperature of below ~46 C°/50 °F while zone 11 for example represents an average lowest temperature of above +5 C°/ +40 °F. For Australia add roughly the number six and this scale can still work in assisting you to determine your outside growing potential. Since frost is a major deciding factor in deciding which plants can grow outside and which not I included this data as a rough reference point to help you in making a more informed decision.

Zone: ~ °C / °F

Zone	~ °C	°F	
11	+ 5	+40	and warmer
10	+ 2	+35	
9	- 4	+25	
8	- 9	+15	
7	- 15	+ 5	
6	- 20	- 5	
5	- 26	- 15	
4	- 32	-25	
3	- 37	-35	
2	- 43	-45	
1	- 46	-50	and colder

How to maximize the healing properties of your spices

Instead of a traditional index I created the following chart as a new and user-friendly means to 'connect the dots' between illness and potentially therapeutic spices. The top row lists illness categories in alphabetical order. Once you found your point of interest just go down that column and discover the spices, which have reported potential therapeutic benefits in that area. You can also use this chart to find the herbs which have similar properties and combine them in cooking delicious foods for nourishment and to support your health and that of those you love to cook for.

Time proven healing knowledge

Properties discovered in animal tests

Properties discovered in the laboratory

Indicates therapeutic use confirmed in human studies

The following table is based solely on the information used for this particular book. It is by no means a complete list of all the possible ways that spices have continued to serve humanity to produce health, healing, desired level of energy and other purposes.

The majority of international studies used for this publication were published in global peer-reviewed scientific journals and are available at 'the world's largest medical library', The United States National Library of Medicine, National Institute of Health. Other significant scientific research sources were 'The German Commission E' (Monografie der Kommission E), the World Health Organization (WHO) published Guidelines for the Assessment of Herbal Medicine, and the Cuban Ministry for Health research publication, the Therapeutic Guide to Plant and Honey Remedies (Guia Terapeutica Dispensarial de Fitofarmacos y Apifarmacos).

Legend of symbols used in cells: 🕐 = clock glyph, 🐱 = animal-face glyph, △ = triangle glyph, † = small figure glyph.

	Allergy & Soothing Agent	Artery & Vein Health	Arthritis & Ease of Movement	Asthma & Breathe Easy	Bacteria & Immunity	Blood Health	Blood Pressure Ease	Breast Function and Health	Cancer Prevention/Treatment	Caries Prevention	Circulation Enhancement	Cough Reduction
Acacia					🕐🐱†		🐱		🐱			🕐
Anise	🐱			🐱	🕐†			🕐				🕐🐱
Basil				🐱△			🕐†		🐱			
Bush Tea	🕐			🐱△			🕐🐱△		🕐🐱			🕐
Cajuput				🕐🐱△†				△				🕐
Caraway							🐱	△				
Cardamom		△				△		△				
Cayenne			🕐🐱△†	🕐△					🐱△			
Cinnamon				🕐	🕐△	🐱						
Clove				🕐🐱△†		🐱			🐱			
Cocoa		🕐🐱△†		🕐🐱			🕐🐱△†	△	△			🕐🐱
Coconut	🕐	🕐	🕐	🕐	🕐🐱△†				🕐		🕐	
Cumin					△			🕐				
Fennel					🕐			🕐				🕐
Garlic	🕐		🕐	🕐🐱△†	🕐🐱△†	🕐🐱△†	🕐🐱△†		🐱△			
Ginger		🕐🐱	🕐🐱		△			△	△			🕐
Grains of Paradise				🕐🐱△†				🕐				🕐
Myrrh		🕐	🕐🐱△	🕐	🕐🐱△†	🕐			🕐🐱△†			🕐
Nigella	🕐			🐱	🕐†	🕐		🕐	🐱			🕐
Nutmeg			🕐	🕐	△		🕐🐱	🕐🐱		△		
Oregano					🕐△				🕐△			🕐
Rosemary				△		🕐†			🐱△			
Turmeric	🐱△	🕐🐱△†	🕐🐱△†	🐱△	🕐🐱△†	🕐	🕐		🕐🐱△†			

Cholesterol Balance	Cold & Flu Support	Diabetic Ease	Digestive Support - General	--Adenomatous polyposis	--Anal fissure	--Constipation	--Crohn's disease	--Diarrhea	--Flatulence, cramps, bloating	--Gastric ulcers	--Gastrointestinal cancer	
		🕐				👤		🕐 👤				Acacia
	🕐		🕐						🕐 🐱	🕐 🐱		Anise
🐱	🕐		🕐 🐱			🕐		🐱	🕐		🐱	Basil
🕐 🐱	🕐											Bush Tea
🕐							🕐					Cajuput
🐱		🕐 🐱	🕐					🕐		🕐 🐱		Caraway
△			🕐 🐱 △ 👤						🐱	△		Cardamom
△		🕐 △ 👤									🐱	Cayenne
		🐱 △						🕐				Cinnamon
		△	🕐		👤			🕐				Clove
🕐 🐱 △ 👤		🕐 🐱					🕐					Cocoa
🕐 🐱 △ 👤	🕐	🕐	🕐	🕐	🕐	🕐	🕐	🕐	🕐	🕐	🕐	Coconut
🐱		🕐 🐱 △	🕐				🕐	🕐	△		🕐 🐱	Cumin
		🕐 🐱 △ 👤							👤	🐱		Fennel
🕐 🐱 △ 👤		👤								△		Garlic
🕐 🐱		🐱 △	🕐 🐱 △ 👤							🕐 △		Ginger
			🕐				🕐 🐱 △			🕐		Grains of Paradise
🕐	🕐	🕐	🕐				🕐	🕐				Myrrh
	🕐	🕐 🐱	🕐 🐱							🕐 🐱		Nigella
🐱		🕐 △	🕐 🐱			🕐		🕐	🕐			Nutmeg
	🕐	🕐 🐱	🕐					🕐				Oregano
	🕐	△	🕐 △ 👤						🕐 👤			Rosemary
🕐		🕐 🐱 △ 👤	🕐 🐱 △ 👤	🕐 🐱 △ 👤	🕐	🕐	🕐	🕐	🕐	🕐 △ 👤	🕐 🐱 △ 👤	Turmeric

	--Hemorroid Ease	--Inflammatory Bowel Disease	--Ulcerative Colitis	Exhaustion	Fever & Temperature Balance	Fungus Treatment	Heart Tonic & Safe Keeping	Immune Support	Inflammation Reduction	Insect Bite Care	Insomnia Relief	Kidney Health
Acacia	🕐	Δ					☺		🕐			
Anise					Δ		🕐 †		Δ			
Basil		☺		🕐	🕐							
Bush Tea							☺					
Cajuput	🕐					🕐 ☺ Δ †			🕐 Δ			
Caraway												
Cardamom						🕐		Δ				
Cayenne						Δ		🕐 ☺		🕐		
Cinnamon				🕐	🕐	†		🕐 †				
Clove	🕐			🕐		🕐 ☺ Δ †			🕐 ☺ Δ †		†	
Cocoa				🕐			🕐 ☺ Δ †					
Coconut	🕐	🕐	🕐	🕐		🕐 ☺ Δ †	🕐 ☺ Δ †	🕐	🕐			
Cumin				🕐								
Fennel				🕐								
Garlic	🕐 †				🕐	🕐 ☺ Δ †	🕐 ☺ Δ †		🕐 ☺ Δ †			
Ginger				🕐		🕐 ☺ Δ †		🕐	🕐 ☺ Δ †			
Grains of Paradise						🕐		🕐 ☺ Δ †	🕐 ☺ Δ †	🕐		
Myrrh	🕐			🕐		🕐			🕐 ☺ Δ †			
Nigella						🕐	🕐 ☺	🕐	🕐 ☺			☺
Nutmeg					🕐		🕐 ☺	🕐	🕐		🕐	🕐
Oregano		🕐				🕐 Δ	🕐	🕐 ☺	🕐	🕐		
Rosemary						Δ	Δ		🕐 ☺			
Turmeric		🕐 ☺ Δ †	🕐 ☺ Δ †			🕐	🕐 ☺ Δ †	🕐 Δ	🕐 ☺ Δ			🕐

Libido Enhancement (Male)	Libido Enhancement (Female)	Liver Health	Memory Enhancement	Menstruation Modulator	Mood Support	Nausea & Vomiting Care	Nervous System Well Being	Oxidative Stress Reduction	Pain Management	--Headaches	--Lumbago	
		🐱		🕐 △				△				Acacia
	🕐	🕐	🕐		🕐							Anise
			🕐		🕐		🐱					Basil
		🕐 🐱			🕐		🐱 △					Bush Tea
								△	🕐		🕐	Cajuput
												Caraway
🕐	🕐							△				Cardamom
											🧍	Cayenne
🕐 🧍	🕐				🕐			△				Cinnamon
🕐	🕐				🕐		🕐 🐱 △ 🧍	🕐 🐱 △ 🧍		🕐	🕐	Clove
🕐 🧍	🕐 🧍				🕐 🐱 △ 🧍		🕐 🐱 △ 🧍	🕐				Cocoa
🕐	🕐	🕐 🐱 △ 🧍			🕐							Coconut
🕐	🕐	🕐						△				Cumin
		🐱	🐱	🧍	🕐		🐱		🧍			Fennel
🕐	🕐		🕐 🐱					🕐		🕐		Garlic
🕐 🐱	🕐	🕐 🐱 △ 🧍				🕐 🐱 △ 🧍	🐱 △					Ginger
🕐 🐱 △	🕐 🐱 △							🕐 🐱 △ 🧍		🕐		Grains of Paradise
		🕐		🕐			🕐	🕐 🐱 △ 🧍				Myrrh
🕐			🕐					🕐				Nigella
🕐 🐱		🐱	🕐 🐱	🕐	🕐 🐱	🕐		🕐	🕐		🕐	Nutmeg
								△	🕐	🕐	🕐	Oregano
		🕐 🧍		🕐		△		🕐			🕐	Rosemary
		🕐	🕐 🐱 △ 🧍	🕐		🕐 🐱 △ 🧍	🕐 🐱 △	🕐				Turmeric

	Sprains & Strains	Toothaches	Parasite Treatment	Malaria	Schistosomiasis	Radiation Protection	Rheumatism Ease	Skin Health	Spasm & Cramp Relaxation	Strong Bone Building	Tonic	Viral Immunity
Acacia			🕐				🕐					△
Anise									🕐	△	🕐	
Basil			😺	🕐							🕐	△
Bush Tea					🕐		🕐	🕐😺△				
Cajuput	🕐	🕐	🕐				🕐	🕐				🕐
Caraway								🕐				
Cardamom									△			😺
Cayenne			🕐	🕐				🧍				🕐😺△🧍
Cinnamon			🕐	🕐								
Clove	🕐	🕐😺△🧍	🕐									🕐😺△🧍
Cocoa						🧍	🕐🧍					
Coconut			🕐△				🕐				🕐😺△🧍	🕐😺△🧍
Cumin								🕐			🕐	
Fennel									🧍		🕐	
Garlic	🕐		🕐😺△🧍	🕐😺△		🕐😺			🕐		🕐😺△🧍	🕐
Ginger	🕐								🕐		🕐	
Grains of Paradise	🕐😺△🧍		🕐	🕐	🕐		🕐	🕐😺△🧍		🕐😺△🧍	🕐	🕐
Myrrh		🕐	🕐😺△🧍		🕐😺△🧍		🕐	🕐			🕐	🕐
Nigella			🕐😺△		🕐△	😺		🕐	😺	😺		
Nutmeg	🕐	🕐				😺	🕐	🕐	🕐		🕐	
Oregano	🕐	🕐	🕐△	🕐	🕐		🕐	🕐				🕐
Rosemary						😺	🕐🧍	🕐	🕐		🕐	
Turmeric			🕐		🕐😺		🕐	🕐😺△🧍	🕐			🕐

HERBAL GLOSSARY

Tea
Many herbal teas can be bought in stores. They are often packaged in single dose tea bags for one cup and are usually taken as a beverage. The tea bag is placed in a hot cup of water and after dunking it a few times, or after three to five minutes, is ready for consumption. Try to obtain unprocessed, organic herbs in a unbleached tea bags. If you are unsure about the bag material, use a tea strainer. These 'cups of tea' can be beneficial but are usually not as strong in their therapeutic functions as an infusion.

Infusion
An infusion is prepared with a specific therapeutic effect in mind. Approximately 150 -250 ml of boiling water is poured over a specifically prescribed amount of the herb. The container is covered and the medicinal properties are allowed to pass from the plant into the water. After occasionally stirring, ten to fifteen minutes later the infusion is strained and consumed at the desired temperature. Infusions are mostly used for dry or fresh leafy herbs or plant materials.

Decoction
A prescribed amount of an herb is poured into a pot filled with cold water and heated to a boil. After boiling five to ten minutes it is allowed to stand for a while then strained. Decoctions are mostly used for harder parts of plants like roots, barks or branches.

Maceration
In the process of heating, some herbs release unwanted or potentially harmful substances. It has been noted that many of these unwanted substances are less soluble in cold water. A specific amount of cold water is poured over a prescribed dose of an herb and is allowed to sit at room temperature for several hours. Finally the liquid is passed through a strainer and consumed. This method of extraction has the obvious benefits of extracting only desired substances, however, it does not kill germs. The impact of possible germ contamination must be considered in balance with the health benefit of extracting only the desired substance or substances.

Infused Oil
Infused oils are usually used topically to treat various skin conditions. Place one third of a cup of the dried herb in a clean glass jar and pour cold pressed organic olive oil over it until covered. After about five to six hours check to see if the herb has not absorbed the oil completely. Add more oil as needed to assure a liquid medium for the herb. Cover the top of the jar with a clean piece of cotton and use a strong rubber band to hold it in place. The oil and the herb must be allowed to breathe. Place the jar in the sun for a week to ten days so the oil can absorb the active therapeutic substances of the herb. Then strain the contents of the jar, and store the infused oil in a brown glass container with a plastic lid.

Ointments and Creams
The only difference between ointments and creams is that ointments are usually softer in their texture. Both consist of the same ingredients but in different quantities. They are used, like the infused oils, for topical applications to treat skin conditions like inflammations, fungal infections, or minor wound care.

To make one cup of an herbal cream, blend a half a cup of an infused oil, a quarter cup of melted beeswax or cocoa butter, and a quarter cup of coconut oil or cold pressed-organic olive oil.

The best way to get the right consistency is to use an electric mixer. Place the cream or ointment in a plastic jar with a plastic lid. In Cuba creams are made fresh, and used as a weekly supply. Refrigeration increases shelf life significantly. If you notice a change in scent, color, or fungal growth discard the cream, and make a fresh batch.

Poultice
A poultice is basically enough freshly chopped plant material to cover the wound or infected area of the skin. To hold it in place it is usually wrapped with a bandage or sandwiched between two cotton layers while the healing properties begin to work.

Tincture
Tinctures are usually prepared by pouring an approximate eighty proof natural alcohol over the selected dry or fresh herb, then macerated for a period of about six weeks.

Index by Health Concern

Allergy & Soothing Agent
Anise • Bush Tea • Coconut • Garlic • Nigella • Turmeric

Aphrodisiac (female)
Anise • Cardamom • Cinnamon • Clove • Cocoa • Coconut • Cumin • Garlic • Ginger • Grains of Paradise

Aphrodisiac (male)
Cardamom • Cinnamon • Clove • Cocoa • Coconut • Cumin • Garlic • Ginger • Grains of Paradise • Nigella • Nutmeg

Artery & Vein Health
Cardamom • Cocoa • Coconut • Myrrh • Turmeric

Arthritis & Ease of Movement
Cayenne • Coconut • Garlic • Ginger • Myrrh • Nigella • Nutmeg • Turmeric

Asthma & Breathe Easy
Anise • Bush Tea • Cinnamon • Cocoa • Coconut • Garlic • Myrrh • Nigella • Nutmeg • Turmeric

Bacteria & Immunity
Acacia • Anise • Basil • Cajuput • Cayenne • Cinnamon • Clove • Coconut • Cumin • Fennel • Garlic • Ginger • Grains of Paradise • Myrrh • Nigella • Nutmeg • Oregano • Rosemary • Turmeric

Blood Health
Cardamom • Cinnamon • Clove • Garlic • Myrrh • Rosemary • Turmeric

Blood Pressure Ease
Acacia • Basil • Bush Tea • Caraway • Cocoa • Garlic • Nigella • Nutmeg • Turmeric

Breast Function & Health
Anise • Cocoa • Cumin • Fennel • Ginger • Nigella

Cancer Prevention & Treatment
Acacia • Basil • Bush Tea • Cajuput • Caraway • Cardamom • Cayenne • Clove • Cocoa • Coconut • Garlic • Ginger • Grains of Paradise • Myrrh • Nigella • Oregano • Rosemary • Turmeric

Caries Prevention
Nutmeg

Circulation Enhancement
Coconut • Cayenne

Cough Reduction
Acacia • Anise • Bush Tea • Cajuput • Cocoa • Fennel • Ginger • Grains of Paradise • Myrrh • Nigella • Oregano

Cholesterol Balance
Basil • Bush Tea • Cajuput • Caraway • Cardamom • Cayenne • Cocoa • Coconut • Cumin • Garlic • Ginger • Myrrh • Nutmeg • Turmeric

Cold and Flu Support
Anise • Basil • Bush Tea • Coconut • Myrrh • Nigella • Oregano • Rosemary

Diabetic Ease
Acacia • Caraway • Cayenne • Cinnamon • Clove • Cocoa • Coconut • Cumin • Garlic • Ginger • Myrrh • Nigella • Nutmeg • Oregano • Rosemary • Turmeric

Digestive Support – General
Anise • Basil • Caraway • Cardamom • Clove • Coconut • Cumin • Fennel • Ginger • Grains of Paradise • Myrrh • Nigella • Nutmeg • Oregano • Rosemary • Turmeric

Adenomatous polyposis (a type of colon cancer)
Coconut • Turmeric

Anal fissures (tear in anal skin)
Clove • Coconut • Turmeric

Constipation
Acacia • Basil • Coconut • Nutmeg • Turmeric

Crohn's disease (autoimmune affecting the gastrointestinal tract, a from of IBD)
Coconut • Turmeric

Diarrhea
Acacia • Basil • Cajuput • Cocoa • Coconut • Cumin • Grains of Paradise • Myrrh • Nutmeg • Oregano • Turmeric

Flatulence, cramps & bloating
Anise • Basil • Caraway • Cardamom • Cinnamon • Clove • Coconut • Cumin • Fennel • Myrrh • Nutmeg • Rosemary • Turmeric

Gastric ulcers (Stomach ulcers)
Anise • Coconut • Cumin • Fennel • Ginger • Grains of Paradise • Turmeric

Gastrointestinal cancer (other)
Basil • Caraway • Cardamom • Cayenne • Coconut • Cumin • Garlic • Nigella • Turmeric

Hemorrhoid ease (Inflammation of veins in rectum)
Acacia • Cajuput • Clove • Coconut • Garlic • Myrrh

Inflammatory bowel disease (IBD)
Acacia • Basil • Coconut • Oregano • Turmeric

Ulcerative colitis (UC is a from of IBD but can affect other parts of the body)
Coconut • Turmeric

Exhaustion
Basil • Cinnamon • Clove • Cocoa • Coconut • Cumin • Fennel • Ginger • Myrrh

Fever & Temperature Balance
Basil • Cinnamon • Garlic • Nutmeg

Fungus Treatment
Anise • Cajuput • Cayenne • Cinnamon • Clove • Coconut • Garlic • Grains of Paradise • Myrrh • Nigella • Oregano • Rosemary • Turmeric

Heart Tonic & Safe Keeping
Acacia • Cardamom • Cocoa • Coconut • Garlic • Ginger • Nigella • Nutmeg • Oregano • Rosemary • Turmeric

Immune Support
Anise • Bush Tea • Cayenne • Cinnamon • Coconut • Ginger • Grains of Paradise • Nigella • Nutmeg • Oregano • Turmeric

Inflammation Reduction
Acacia • Cajuput • Cardamom • Clove • Coconut • Garlic • Ginger • Grains of Paradise • Myrrh • Nigella • Nutmeg • Oregano • Rosemary • Turmeric

Insect Bites Care
Anise • Cayenne • Clove • Grains of Paradise • Oregano

Insomnia Relief
Nutmeg

Kidney Health
Nigella • Nutmeg • Turmeric

Liver Health
Acacia • Anise • Bush Tea • Coconut • Cumin • Fennel • Ginger • Myrrh • Nutmeg • Rosemary • Turmeric

Memory Enhancement
Fennel • Garlic • Nutmeg • Turmeric

Menstruation Modulator
Anise • Fennel • Myrrh • Nigella • Nutmeg • Rosemary • Turmeric

Mood Support
Acacia • Anise • Basil • Bush Tea • Cocoa • Fennel • Nutmeg

Nausea & Vomiting Care
Basil • Cinnamon • Clove • Coconut • Ginger • Nutmeg

Nervous System Well Being
Rosemary • Turmeric

Oxidative Stress Reduction
Acacia • Basil • Bush Tea • Cajuput • Cinnamon • Clove • Cocoa • Cumin • Fennel • Ginger • Myrrh • Nutmeg • Oregano • Turmeric

Pain Management - General
Cajuput • Cardamom • Clove • Cocoa • Fennel • Garlic • Grains of Paradise • Myrrh • Nigella • Nutmeg • Oregano • Rosemary • Turmeric

Headaches
Clove • Oregano

Lumbago
Cajuput • Cayenne • Clove • Garlic • Grains of Paradise • Nutmeg • Oregano • Rosemary

Sprains & strains
Cajuput • Clove • Garlic • Ginger • Grains of Paradise • Nutmeg • Oregano

Toothaches
Cajuput • Clove • Myrrh • Nutmeg • Oregano

Parasite Treatment - General
Acacia • Basil • Cajuput • Cayenne • Cinnamon • Clove • Coconut • Garlic • Grains of Paradise • Myrrh • Nigella • Oregano • Turmeric

Malaria
Basil • Cayenne • Cinnamon • Garlic • Grains of Paradise • Oregano

Schistosomiasis
Grains of Paradise • Myrrh • Nigella • Oregano • Turmeric

Radiation Protection
Bush Tea • Cocoa • Garlic • Nigella • Nutmeg • Rosemary

Rheumatism Ease
Cajuput • Cayenne • Grains of Paradise • Myrrh • Nutmeg • Oregano • Rosemary • Turmeric

Skin Health
Acacia • Bush Tea • Cajuput • Cocoa • Coconut • Grains of Paradise • Myrrh • Nigella • Nutmeg • Oregano • Rosemary • Turmeric

Spasms & Cramp Relaxation
Anise • Bush Tea • Caraway • Cardamom • Cumin • Fennel • Garlic • Ginger • Nigella • Rosemary • Turmeric

Strong Bone Building
Anise • Grains of Paradise • Nigella

Tonic
Anise • Basil • Coconut • Cumin • Fennel • Garlic • Ginger • Grains of Paradise • Myrrh • Nutmeg • Rosemary

Viral Immunity
Acacia • Basil • Cajuput • Cardamom • Cayenne • Clove • Coconut • Garlic • Grains of Paradise • Myrrh • Oregano • Turmeric

www.ingramcontent.com/pod-product-compliance
Lightning Source LLC
Chambersburg PA
CBHW031205270326
41931CB00006B/422